Analgesic Drugs

J. PARKHOUSE
MA, MD, MSc, FFARCS.
Professor of Anaesthetics

B. J. PLEUVRY
BPharm, MSc, PhD, MPS
Research Associate in Anaesthetics

J. M. H. REES
MSc, PhD
Senior Lecturer in Pharmacology

Departments of Anaesthetics and Pharmacology
University of Manchester

BLACKWELL

SCIENTIFIC PUBLICATIONS

OXFORD   LONDON   EDINBURGH

MELBOURNE

© 1979 Blackwell Scientific Publications
Osney Mead, Oxford, OX2 0EL
8 John Street, London, W1N 2ES
9 Forrest Road, Edinburgh, EH1 2QH
P.O. Box 9, North Balwyn, Victoria, Australia

First published 1979

British Library Cataloguing in Publication Data

Parkhouse, James
    Analgesic drugs.
    1. Analgesics
    I. Title   II. Pleuvry, B J   III. Rees, J M
    615'.783   RM319

ISBN 0-632-00433-9

Distributed in U.S.A. by
Blackwell Mosby Book Distributors
11830 Westline Industrial Drive
St. Louis, Missouri 63141
and in Canada by
Blackwell Mosby Book Distributors
86 Northline Road, Toronto
Ontario, M4B 3E5

Set by Santype Ltd, Salisbury
Printed in Great Britain at the Alden Press, Oxford
and bound at Kemp Hall Bindery

Analgesic Drugs

Contents

Preface

This book is a review of the pharmacology and therapeutic usefulness of drugs commonly used for the relief of pain. Particular emphasis has been placed on recent advances in mechanisms of analgesic drug activity and the design of clinical trials for this class of compounds. Detailed discussion of individual agents has been limited to those which have achieved widespread popularity as analgesic agents. Drugs used mainly for their anti-inflammatory properties are not included.

While the book is intended for undergraduates and for post-graduate revision, it is hoped that it will also be useful as a basis for more extensive studies in this field.

Chapter 1 · Pain Mechanisms and the Nature of Pain

Since analgesic drugs are, by definition, those given to relieve pain it is appropriate to begin with a brief general description of the nature of pain and its perception. For a more detailed account of current views on the neuro-physiology of pain mechanisms the reader is particularly recommended to refer to the excellent chapter by Bowsher (1977). Other symposia and reviews dealing with relevant work on pain mechanisms are those of Payne and Burt (1972), Bonica (1974), Nakahama (1975) and Bonica and Albe-Fessard (1977).

Following Muller's theory of nerve specificity, von Frey (1895) described four specific types of cutaneous receptors, one of which he believed to subserve pain. The opposite view, that of functional non-specificity of such nerve endings, was put forward by Lele and Weddell (1959). More recent evidence indicates that three categories of cutaneous receptors can be identified: mechanoreceptors, thermoreceptors and nociceptors (Iggo 1976). There is also evidence for the existence of specific visceral and muscle nociceptors (Iggo 1972). Mechanoreceptors and thermoreceptors respond at a low threshold of stimulation, and impulses are transmitted by way of large nerve fibres to the posterior columns of the spinal cord and thence via the medial lemniscus. There are, however, collateral fibres to the substantia gelatinosa capable of modifying transmission at this point. Pain cannot be explained simply on the basis of high intensity stimulation of receptors which subserve other modalities of sensation; specific nociceptors, which appear to show some differential sensitivity to heat and pressure, have a high response threshold. Transmission is by way of small (1–5 μm) myelinated fibres (A delta) and unmyelinated C fibres (0·5–1 μm), passing to the dorsal horn and substantia gelatinosa respectively and then upwards in the anterolateral quadrant of the opposite side of the spinal cord. Pain and hyperalgesia may be elicited 'indirectly" when pathology or trauma causes

1

loss of insulation betweeen adjacent fibres in a nerve trunk so that activity in low-threshold fibres can cross-excite fibres otherwise activated only at a higher threshold (Zotterman 1972).

Nociceptors may well, in fact, be chemoreceptors. Since the first studies of Sir Thomas Lewis, a considerable literature has grown up around the concept of pain-producing substances which may be liberated as a result of trauma or disease (Keele & Armstrong 1964). The potential role of various compounds, including histamine, 5-hydroxytryptamine, bradykinin and other related peptides, is reviewed by Werle (1972). More recently prostaglandins have been studied in this context (Vane 1971) and their relationship to the possible mechanism of action of mild analgesics is discussed in Chapter 4.

The initial sensation of acute skin trauma is a transient, sharp, pricking pain, described as fast pain and mediated by myelinated fibres. The more unpleasant and more prolonged, burning type of pain (slow pain) which may follow fast pain or result from other causes of tissue damage is mediated by unmyelinated C fibres. Visceral pain and pain from deep somatic structures (also transmitted by C fibre activity) is characteristically not localized, aching in character and often associated with autonomic disturbance such as nausea. It is 'fast' pain which is characteristically conveyed along the classical pathway through the spino–thalamic tract to those thalamic nuclei which project directly into the cortex. Unmyelinated C fibres, which predominate in the peripheral nerves, transmit via the substantia gelatinosa and the spino-reticular fibres of the anterolateral quadrant of the cord to the brain stem reticular neurones and intralaminar nuclei of the thalamus of both sides. The primary importance of these reticular pathways must be appreciated. Bowsher (1977) makes the point that, although most research has been concerned with pricking pain, it is pathological pain of the 'slow' variety with which clinicians are invariably concerned.

Although the spino–thalamic and spino–recticular pathways are largely independent, there are communications at thalamic and other levels, and projection not only from thalamus to the post-central gyrus of the cortex, but to the hypothalamus, corpus striatum and limbic system. Hence there are complex interconnections capable of eliciting respiratory, cardiovascular, vocal, autonomic and other involuntary accompaniments of pain perception. Pain may originate centrally (thalamic pain) when cerebral tumour or softening affects the ventro–caudal nucleus of the thalamus.

The posterior horn and substantia gelatinosa are points of convergence of many incoming fibres of differing diameter from body surface, deep and visceral sources. Again intercommunication provides a variety of possible explanations for referred pain, reflex muscle spasm and associated phenomena. A detailed account of the classical work on referred pain is given by Bonica (1953) and the localization of referral of pain of musculo-skeletal origin is reviewed by Kellgren (1969). Reference has been made to the influence of large fibre activity, via collaterals, on the substantia gelatinosa. The additional influence of descending impulses must also be remembered. It is easy to understand how the balance of power between these various influences should have led to the concept of a 'gate' within the substantia gelatinosa (Melzak & Wall 1965), and how low-threshold stimulation of large fibres by rubbing the skin and other methods of 'counter-irritation', or the application of an external nerve stimulator, may produce relief.

It is worth emphasizing at this stage that pain arising along the course of the nerve pathway may be indistinguishable from pain arising at the natural peripheral termination of the affected fibres. Pain may appear to arise in the more distal part of a limb which no longer exists, as in phantom pain; even angina may 'radiate' to a left arm amputated many years previously (Cohen & Jones 1943).

The pain pathways described above involve innumerable synapses where chemical transmission of impulses takes place. The identity of the transmitter substances involved in these pathways has been the subject of intensive research. Some of the evidence for and against various biogenic amines having a role in pain perception, analgesia and, more specifically, the analgesia produced by narcotic analgesic agents has been reviewed by Clouet (1971) and Sewell and Spencer (1977). From this work it is clear that reaction to pain and modification of analgesic activity does not depend upon a single monoamine. On balance it would seem that tryptaminergic and cholinergic systems tend to lower appreciation of pain, while dopaminergic systems enhance pain perception.

More recently the situation has been further complicated by studies directed towards the involvement of a variety of endogenous peptides in pain transmission and analgesia. A possible role of Sub-

Table 1. Analgesic testing methods in the experimental animal

	Species	Comments
A. *Thermal methods*		
Tail flick test (D'Amour & Smith 1941)	Mouse/rat	Minimal tissue damage even when used repeatedly on the same animal. Will not predict the potency of narcotic antagonist analgesics or weak non-narcotic analgesics. End-point is a reflex response.
Hot plate test (Woolfe & Macdonald, 1944)	Mouse/rat	As above. Competent, trained observers are necessary to obtain reproducible results.
B. *Mechanical methods*		
Tail pressure (Haffner 1929)	Rat/mouse	Squeak end-point. There is a danger of tissue damage which would make repeat measurements impossible. Lack of precision in the stimulus and end-point. Not useful for screening narcotic antagonist analgesics.
Skin pressure	Any	As above.
Distension of hollow viscera (Eddy 1932)	Any	As above.
Inflamed paw (Randall and Selitto 1957)	Usually rat	Detects narcotic and non-narcotic analgesics. Increase in pain threshold may be due to anti-inflammatory action rather than true analgesia.

C. *Chemical methods*

Writhing test (Collier 1964)	Mouse/rat	Detects all types of analgesics, but also gives positive results for compounds not normally considered as analgesics, e.g. antihistamine agents.

D. *Electrical stimulation*

Tooth pulp stimulation	Dog, rabbit, guinea pig	Preparation of animals is time consuming. Conditioning occurs rapidly especially in the dog (i.e. the animal responds to the experimental set up rather than to the pulp stimulation). It is difficult to obtain reproducible results and painful stimulation of the teeth can lead to hyperirritability which extends for months.
Electrical stimulation of other parts of the body	Any	Resistance of tissues is variable and not easy to control. Sensitivity is low and the response to a given drug varies with age, sex, strain and many other factors.
Flinch–jump procedure (Evans 1962)	Rat	Behavioral response. Poor correlation between drug activity in this test and actual analgesic activity in man. However, nalorphine-like drugs and non-narcotic analgesics can be detected.

stance P as a transmitter of noxious stimuli in the spinal cord has been proposed (Jessell & Iversen 1977) and the discovery of endogenous morphine–like peptides in both the brain and spinal cord has enhanced our understanding of the mechanisms of opiate actions significantly (Chapter 2).

Perception of pain

Interpretation of pain and its significance to the patient are at least as important as the mechanisms determining the arrival of the causal impulses within the central nervous system. As pointed out already, the origin of painful impulses generated at various points along the nervous pathway to the cortex may be falsely interpreted. It remains to be said that 'pain', as a human concept, exists only in the brain or, if such terminology is preferred, in the mind. To say, therefore, that a patient's pain is 'all in the mind' is to do no more than state the obvious. To say that it is 'psychological' or 'psychogenic', although medically and scientifically imprecise, may give a better indication of the probable point of its primary generation. However, in treating pain, the central nature of the sensation itself and its consequences, regardless of where they may seem to arise or be seen to appear, must be appreciated at all times. The clinician's attitude to a patient with pain should be rather like Bertrand Russell's (1959) attitude to our knowledge of the external world, when he wrote: "I may illustrate how I differ from most philosophers by quoting the title of an article by Mr. H. Hudson in *Mind* of April, 1956. His article is entitled, 'Why we cannot witness or observe what goes on "in our heads"'. What I maintain is that we *can* witness or observe what goes on in our heads, and that we cannot witness or observe anything else at all".

In connection with this point, it should be remembered that some methods of assessing analgesic drug action, such as the tail flick test in mice, can be seen even in decapitated animals (Keats 1969). This is a sufficient comment on the gap that can exist between an objective end-point indicating pharmacological action, and the conscious human feeling that we call pain. Nevertheless, experimental methods are of great value in the detection of possible analgesic effect and in the screening and further study of analgesic compounds.

The usefulness of analgesic testing methods in the experimental animal depends on their ability to predict the analgesic activity of a given compound in man. Some of the more important methods are listed in Table 1. All can detect the actions of morphine-like drugs and most can predict with fair accuracy relative potency ratios for these drugs in man. However, none of the tests listed can predict the analgesic potency of the narcotic antagonist analgesics. Indeed only a few of the tests can even detect activity in this class of drug. It may be that the narcotic antagonist analgesics exhibit analgesic activity only in man, since even the monkey fails to response to nalorphine.

More detailed reviews of methods of assessing pain in animals can be found in Beecher (1957), Collier (1964) and Winter (1965).

Further information must be obtained in human volunteers before analgesic drugs are put into general clinical use. Many methods of eliciting pain for experimental purposes have been described, and serious efforts have been made to standardize the appropriate techniques. Probably the most widely used methods have been the application of radiant heat in a controlled manner to a suitably prepared area of skin (Hardy *et al.* 1949); 'algesimetry', or the application of graded pressure to the skin, usually over the tibia (Head & Holmes 1912a, b, Clutton-Brock 1964, Thorpe 1966); and ischaemic pain produced by requiring the subject to exercise the arm while the blood supply is occluded, (e.g. Parkhouse *et al.* 1960). Algesimetry and ischaemic pain are certainly both capable of producing useful results, but the experimenter must be prepared to induce severe pain (and the volunteer subjects must be prepared to endure it) in order to ensure that active drugs can be distinguished from placebos (Smith *et al.* 1966).

Since this book is concerned primarily with the pharmacology of analgesic drugs and their clinical applicability, further discussion of methods of evaluation will be confined to controlled clinical trials (Chapter 6).

Chapter 2 · Narcotic Analgesics and Antagonists
I. Mechanisms of action and general pharmacology

Drugs alter brain activity by interfering with chemical transmission in the central nervous system. Whilst the complexity of chemical transmission in the brain is beyond its own understanding, our knowledge of chemical transmission in the peripheral nervous system is considerable, as is our understanding of the ways in which drugs can interfere with it. Using these peripheral mechanisms as precedents, it is believed that drugs interfere with central chemical transmission in similar ways. There are analogies with drugs which mimic the actions of a neurotransmitter, those that interfere with its neuronal release, antagonize its pre- and post-synaptic actions, prevent its uptake, or interfere with its synthesis or metabolism. In these terms we can explain up to a point the mechanisms of many centrally acting drugs including the phenothiazines, the tricyclic antidepressants and the hallucinogens. These drugs interfere more or less selectively with certain neurotransmitters.

The narcotic analgesics have selective central actions, and it has always been assumed that they too interfere with a specific neurotransmitter, but the nature of this transmitter has remained unknown until recently.

In years to come, writers on this topic will be able to preface an account of the pharmacology of morphine with a description of the central physiological systems with which it interacts. In just the same way today, an account of the pharmacology of the antiparkinson drugs may be prefaced with an account of cholinergic and dopaminergic control of central motor co-ordination and their imbalance in disease, thereby providing a rational approach to its drug treatment.

Our current knowledge of the physiology relevant to morphine is, however, unclear. Whilst this aspect is dealt with later (p. 29) some mention of it is made here in which context the more orthodox account of the pharmacology of morphine which follows may be considered.

The first indication that morphine selectively interferes with chemical transmission was found, predictably, in the more accessible peripheral nervous system.

Electrical stimulation of the postganglionic parasympathetic nerves supplying the guinea pig ileum causes a release of endogenous acetylcholine, and the muscle contracts. Application of morphine inhibits these contractions, and this inhibition was shown to be due to the prevention of release of acetylcholine (Cox & Weinstock 1966). This is a presynaptic action of morphine.

A morphine 'receptor' on the nerve ending was postulated, and its similarity with those in the central nervous system was noted since potency ratios between morphine derivatives were the same in both cases (Kosterlitz, Lord & Watt 1973). A diagram showing this unusual correlation is shown in Fig. 2.1. In addition it had been shown that naloxone antagonized this peripheral action of morphine just as it will antagonize the central actions of this drug (Kosterlitz & Watt 1968).

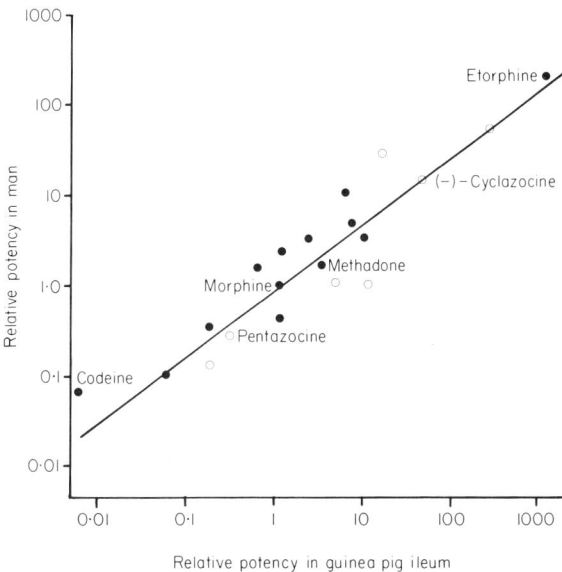

Fig. 2.1. The correlation of the potencies of opiates to inhibit contractions of the guinea pig ileum *in vitro*, and their potencies as analgesics in man. The correlation applies to both pure agonists (●), and partial agonists (○). For clarity only a limited selection of drugs is identified. For details see Kosterlitz (1975), and Kosterlitz and Waterfield (1975).

This observation precipitated much speculation that morphine might act similarly on the central nervous system by preventing acetylcholine release. In retrospect such a precise explanation was unrealistic since this peripheral action is almost unique. For instance, morphine has no effect on the release of acetylcholine from most other postganglionic parasympathetic nerve endings (e.g. to the heart), and there is little evidence to show that it affects acetylcholine release to the ileum in many species other than the guinea pig.

Thus such a simple explanation could not explain the diverse actions of morphine. In addition evidence had accumulated that morphine interfered with other transmitters in the central nervous system—noradrenaline, dopamine and most notably 5-hydroxytryptamine (see Clouet 1971, Kosterlitz, Collier & Villarreal 1972).

Some workers even dismissed the peripheral 'model' as a coincidence unrelated to central mechanisms of action.

The next step in this fascinating elucidation of mechanism of action was again observed in the periphery (Henderson, Hughes & Kosterlitz 1972). They demonstrated that morphine also depressed the release of transmitter from the postganglionic sympathetic nerve endings supplying the vas deferens of the mouse. In this instance the transmitter is noradrenaline. Again, this is a highly selective effect of morphine, since the drug does not inhibit noradrenaline release at most other sympathetic nerve endings.

The implication was therefore made that morphine's ability to inhibit transmitter release was a characteristic of the nerve ending independent of its location in the autonomic nervous system, or of the transmitter that was released.

Any theories (and there were many of them) which associated morphine's action specifically with a single known transmitter system were dispelled by the work of Kuhar, Pert and Snyder (1973). Using radioactively labelled morphine derivatives they were able to map out specific binding sites for opiates throughout the brain. These specific binding sites are presumed to indicate the presence of opiate receptors. Their distribution is shown in Table 2.1.

The important conclusion drawn from this work was that the distribution of opiate receptors in the brain differed from those of any known transmitter.

Since that important paper, our understanding as to how morphine could produce its various effects has leapt forward with the identification of the long-suspected chemicals in the brain with

Table 2.1. The distribution of stereospecific opiate binding sites in monkey brain. For full details see Kuhar, Pert and Snyder (1973).

Stereospecific opiate binding (fmol/mg protein)	Region of monkey central nervous system
> 30	Anterior and posterior amygdala Periaqueductal gray matter
> 20	Medial, anterior & posterior Hypothalamus Medial thalamus
> 10	Caudate nucleus Interpeduncular nucleus Hippocampus Frontal pole Putamen Superior temporal gyrus Superior colliculi
> 5	Spinal cord (gray matter) Raphe area Lateral thalamus Globus pallidus Medial & inferior temporal gyrus Inferior colliculi Floor of 4th ventricle Lower medulla Mammillary bodies

morphine-like activity and furthermore with the evidence for these being neuronal in origin. We know some of their actions, but their physiological significance is unclear. The most recent developments in our understanding of morphine's pharmacology are described at the end of this section.

The description of the actions of morphine which follows may be considered in the light of our knowledge of the locations of morphine receptors in the central nervous system.

The pharmacology of narcotic analgesics and their antagonists

Two terms are commonly used to refer to morphine derivatives, the *narcotic* and *opiate* analgesics. The term narcotic was originally used to distinguish these analgesics from the antipyretic analgesics since the former cause narcosis, a state of stupor and insensibility. On the other hand the term opiate means contained in or derived from opium. Neither term is therefore satisfactory since some 'narcotic' analgesics do not cause narcosis, and the relationship between some 'opiates' and opium is very distant.*

Nevertheless both terms are widely used, and both are adopted in this summary of their pharmacology.

The clinical use, prediction of side effects and contraindications of narcotic analgesics depend on two basic properties of morphine and its pharmacological analogues.

1. The derivatives of morphine can act either as agonists or as antagonists.
2. The narcotic agonists have selective depressant and excitatory actions on various areas in the central nervous system.

Agonist and antagonist ratios

The convenient term 'agonist', commonly used by pharmacologists, refers to a physiological chemical or a drug which produces a primary effect at a receptor, which effect can be reduced selectively by an antagonist.

Morphine is a pure agonist, producing the well-known range of effects—analgesia, respiratory depression, cough suppression, sedation, vomiting and constipation.

Naloxone is a pure opiate antagonist, competitively antagonizing the actions of a pure agonist.

These two type substances are called 'pure' since morphine has no clinically detectable antagonist activity, and naloxone has no detectable agonist activity, i.e. the injection of large doses of naloxone into a control subject will produce negligible effects.

All morphine derivatives fall within this spectrum between pure agonist and pure antagonist. The ratios of agonist to antagonist activities are summarized in Fig. 2.2.

The most important intermediate drug is pentazocine. Pentazocine possesses both agonist and antagonist activities, a most confusing property. When given alone pentazocine will produce typical agonist effects similar to those listed for morphine. On the other

---

* Recently, the grammatically more correct, though uglier, term *opioid* has been adopted by many researchers.

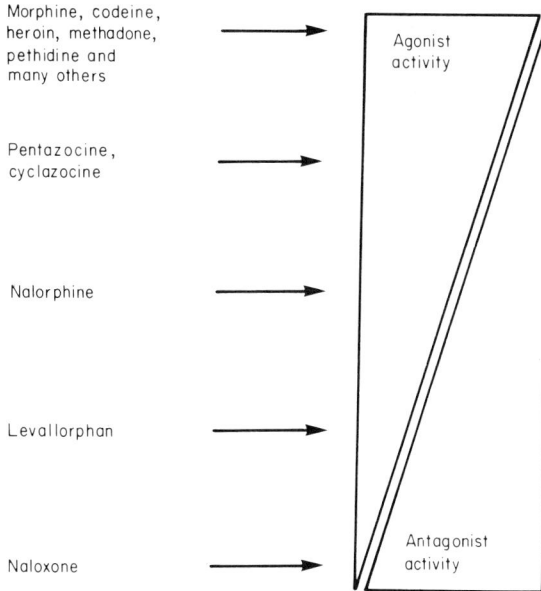

Morphine, codeine, heroin, methadone, pethidine and many others

Pentazocine, cyclazocine

Nalorphine

Levallorphan

Naloxone

Agonist activity

Antagonist activity

Fig. 2.2.

hand, if it is given to a subject following injection of a pure agonist, its antagonist activity will be apparent. Such a drug is known as a partial agonist, or as a narcotic antagonist analgesic.

The significance of these ratios is considerable, and the figure should be consulted at intervals during the text. At this early stage two points are made. Firstly, there are specific antidotes to narcotic agonist poisoning. Secondly, there are some crucial differences between the characteristics of pure agonists and agonists which also possess antagonist activity, e.g. morphine compared with pentazocine.

Depressant and excitatory actions

Morphine produces a wide range of selective depressant effects (e.g. respiratory depression) and excitatory effects (e.g. vomiting). The term excitation is used here to describe both direct stimulation and depression of inhibition.

Although the net effect is nearly always depression, the opiates differ from other CNS depressants such as the barbiturates in that their effects are *selective*.

This selectivity of action is well illustrated by consideration of the actions of morphine on physiological functions which are primarily controlled from within one small area of the brain stem at the level of the medulla oblongata.

The locations of some major physiological control centres in this plane are shown in Fig. 2.3.

Within this plane morphine will depress respiration, yet has no effect on the anatomically and physiologically integrated vasomotor centre. It will stimulate the superficial chemosensitive trigger zone of the vomiting centre, yet subsequently depress the vomiting centre itself. It will stimulate the vagal nucleus, yet depress the cough centre.

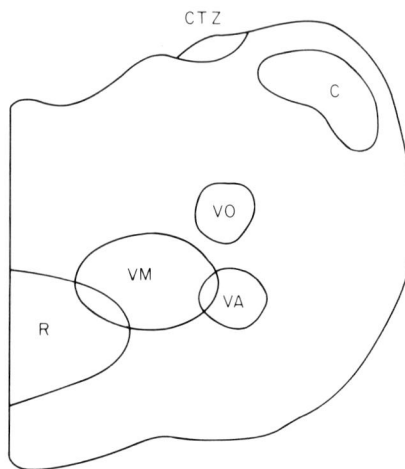

Fig. 2.3 Unilateral section through the medulla oblongata showing the approximate locations of the respiratory centres (**R**), vasomotor centre (**VM**), vagal nucleus (**VA**), vomiting centre (**VO**), cough centre (**C**) and chemosensitive trigger zone of the vomiting reflex (**CTZ**).

In addition, this selectivity is further illustrated in the existence of morphine derivatives which retain some actions but not others. For instance apomorphine (p. 62) will stimulate the chemosensitive trigger zone yet has little effect elsewhere. Dextromethorphan suppresses the cough centre, yet has no effect on the closely integrated respiratory centres.

Central agonist actions

Depressant actions: analgesia, sedation (which can progress to anaesthesia), cough suppression.

Excitatory actions: euphoria, hallucinations, convulsions, release of ADH, miosis, vomiting.

The net effect is generally depression, but the likelihood of excitatory manifestations varies within the drug group. For instance, one is more likely to see excitatory effects after the derivatives of codeine and pethidine than after morphine or heroin.

Analgesia

The definition of pain favoured by this writer is that of Bishop (quoted in Beecher 1957):

'Pain is what the subject says hurts'.

Thus, there are two components of pain which may be targets for analgesic drugs. First, there are those neuroanatomical pathways known to be responsible for the transmission, integration and interpretation of pain impulses. Secondly, there is the subjective reaction of the individual to the stimulus. Narcotic analgesics act on both components, the ratio being dependent on circumstance.

Despite the wide range of morphine's actions, analgesia will be produced at doses which cause insignificant clinical side effects. Prolonged dull pain is more susceptible to morphine than is intermittent sharp pain, thereby suggesting a selective effect on one of the two major pain pathways. But the distinction is not absolute since with higher doses, sharp pain, for example that of biliary colic, will be relieved.

The distinction between an effect on pain threshold and the subsequent reaction to pain is difficult. Experimentally-produced pain differs from pathological pain in that a subject exposed to experimental pain knows that at the end of the experiment the pain will cease. His reaction to it will therefore differ from that of a patient suffering from pathological pain who knows that the pain will return, and also that the pain may be indicative of serious disease.

Whilst there is no doubt that morphine can alter the pain threshold, in clinical use the major component of its analgesic action is an altered attitude to pain. Patients will say that the pain can still be perceived, but that their reaction to it has changed—it does not matter so much.

This altered attitude to pain caused by morphine is closely linked with its euphoriant action.

In patients with pathological pain morphine causes *euphoria*, a feeling of well-being. It is assumed that this euphoriant action is the major component of its analgesic action. In this context it is particularly interesting to note that in pain-free volunteers morphine is as likely to cause dysphoria—a feeling of being generally miserable.

Whilst an altered attitude to pain remains the more important component, an effect on pain threshold does exist. Some morphine derivatives, particularly amongst the narcotic antagonist analgesics, possess analgesic activity, yet they do not cause euphoria.

The site of analgesic action has variously been ascribed to spinal, brain stem, mid brain and cortical regions. Whilst no precise conclusions can be drawn, two points may be made.

Firstly it is significant that a high density of opiate binding sites are in the Limbic System (p. 11). This is compatible with the well-known actions of opiates on mood, and the involvement of mood change in their analgesic action.

Secondly, in animal studies, central microinjections of opiates have shown most sensitive analgesic sites in structures surrounding the third ventricle in rats (Jacquet & Lajtha 1973) and in monkeys (Pert & Yaksh 1974), and regions near the floor of the fourth ventricle in rabbits (Hertz, Albus, Metys, Shubert & Teschemacher 1970). Van Ree (1977) showed that analgesia could be caused by morphine following injection into a wide range of brain sites in rats. Correlations between these brain stem regions, the distribution of opiate binding sites, and pain pathways have been made by several authors (e.g. Pert 1975).

Differences between individual opiate agonists are reviewed later. In general they differ in four ways.

Firstly, they differ in terms of potency. In this context potency means maximum possible effect rather than weight for weight potency. Of clinically used drugs, heroin is the most potent, then in decreasing order, morphine (and many others), pethidine, dihydrocodeine, codeine and dextropropoxyphene.

Secondly, they differ in terms of the incidence of undesirable side effects accompanying a given degree of analgesia. For instance there is no clinical value of parenteral codeine. In high doses it can cause the same degree of analgesia as 10 mg morphine, but the high incidence of side effects precludes the use of such a dose. Vomiting is a common undesirable side effect of opiates. Sedation may or may not be desirable dependent on clinical circumstance.

Thirdly, they differ in oral efficacy. Morphine, by virtue of its relatively polar (water soluble) structure is poorly absorbed from the gastrointestinal tract. In contrast some of its derivatives, for example dextromoramide, are well absorbed.

Lastly, they differ in their durations of action. Those drugs used in the technique of neuroleptanalgesia (e.g. fentanyl, p. 45) have a very short duration of action, whilst some other derivatives maintain analgesia for up to 6 hours.

These important differences are covered in the section on the individual agents (p. 42 *et seq.*).

Respiratory depression

Whilst normal therapeutic doses of morphine cause little respiratory embarrassment, respiratory depression will always accompany analgesia, and the same degree of analgesia will be accompanied by the same degree of respiratory depression, irrespective of the pure agonist used, whether a mixture of agonist and antagonist has been given, or the degree of tolerance (Lasagna 1964, Lambertsen 1966, Brown 1971). This unusual correlation between two distinct physiological systems extends to the partial agonists such as pentazocine (Dyrberg, Henningsen & Johansen 1967).

The factors controlling respiratory rate are the main target for respiratory depression, and this may be variably compensated by changes in tidal volume. Arterial Pco_2 rises.

In experimental animals and in man the respiratory depression is accompanied by a decrease in the sensitivity of the brain stem respiratory centres to the stimulant action of CO_2. Thus as Pco_2 rises the elevated threshold is reached and breathing occurs. The subsequent irregular, gasping respiration is characteristic of narcotic analgesic poisoning, and has been interpreted as 'pharmacological decerebration' (Orkin, Egge & Rovenstine 1955).

In addition there is an indifference to respiration: a patient may breathe if so instructed (Jaffe & Martin 1975).

The site of the respiratory depressant action is unknown. Whilst evidence of decreased CO_2 sensitivity is not in doubt, attempts to demonstrate direct depression of medullary respiratory centres have met with variable results (cf. Florez, McCarthy & Borison 1968, Pentiah, Reilly & Borison 1966).

The distribution of opiate binding sites in the CNS shows some to be in the floor of the fourth ventricle (close to the CO_2 sensing elements), and in the limbic system (known to be involved in the considerable voluntary control of respiration).

It seems likely that respiratory depression is due to actions both low in the medulla and in the mid brain.

However striking this respiratory depression may be, and it is the root cause of death in opiate poisoning, man can tolerate the consequences of severe respiratory depression when it has been produced by an opiate much better than when it has been caused by a non-specific central depressant such as barbiturates.

In the latter case respiratory depression is accompanied by severe cardiovascular depression, in the former there is negligible vasomotor depression. A comparison between the doses of the two drug groups which cause severe respiratory depression, and their LD 50 values is striking (Hunter, Pleuvry & Rees 1968).

Cough suppression (Antitussive activity)

A most important theme has become apparent in the account of opiate actions so far, that being the role of subjective drug effects (in pain perception, and in the more unlikely respiratory control). Again it is interesting that, whilst there is no doubt that opiates suppress coughing, the reported relief of patients does not always correlate with decreased incidence of coughing (Sevelius, McCoy & Colmore 1971).

Amongst the agents included in antitussive preparations, the derivatives of morphine are the only agents that actively depress the cough centre.

Since coughing involves forced expiration, it is not surprising that selective respiratory depressants such as morphine should be effective antitussive agents. What is surprising is that whilst attempts to separate the analgesic and respiratory depressant actions of opiates have met with no success, both quantitative and qualitative separation between antitussive and analgesic activities has been achieved. Quantitative separation may be achieved by structural manipulation of the opiate molecule.

If the structure of morphine is considered (Fig. 2.4), the important substituent is that on the benzene ring—in the case of morphine the phenolic hydroxyl group. As a general rule, the larger the substituent in the equivalent position, the more selective will be the antitussive agent. In this way, pethidine (R=H) is a weak antitussive. Morphine (R=OH) is an effective agent, whilst codeine (R=OCH$_3$) is a useful antitussive at sub-analgesic doses. Heroin (R=O·CO·CH$_3$) is the most potent antitussive agent (though its use as such is to be discouraged), and pholcodeine, which has a very large substituent is an effective antitussive agent yet has negligible analgesic activity.

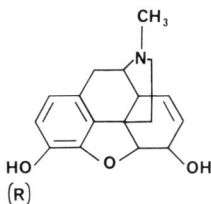

Fig. 2.4. Structure of morphine.

Curiously, qualitative separation between these two actions has been achieved.

Emphasis has been made that the narcotic analgesics are structurally specific drugs in which small changes in structure can lead to large changes in pharmacological activity. It is a characteristic of such drugs that they display stereospecificity—pharmacological activity residing in only one optical isomer. In the case of the opiates, activity normally resides in the l (−) series (equivalent to the absolute configuration of D-morphine). Surprisingly, antitussive activity is retained in some of the d (+) isomers.

Hence dextromethorphan which is an effective antitussive agent (roughly equipotent with codeine), yet possesses virtually no other central activity. It is one of the most selective centrally acting drugs.

Emetic action

Nausea and vomiting are common undesirable side effects of the narcotic analgesics. The mechanism of action is by direct stimulation of the chemosensitive trigger zone of the area postrema in the floor of the fourth ventricle (Wang & Glaviano 1954).

Labyrinthine stimulation increases the incidence of vomiting, it being rare in the supine patient, but relatively high (15 per cent) in the ambulatory subject. Pethidine, which has a higher incidence of excitatory actions, is more likely to cause vomiting than is morphine due to sensitization of the labyrinths (Gutner, Gould & Batterman 1952).

In addition to stimulation of the chemosensitive trigger zone, opiates can subsequently *depress* the deeper lying vomiting centre (Wang 1963). Perhaps because of different rates of blood supply this is why, if vomiting is going to occur following injection of an opiate, it will occur soon after injection. Because of the later depression of the vomiting centre the subsequent risk of vomiting is less.

Apomorphine is a relatively selective emetic in man, lacking most of the other characteristic actions of morphine. Of great interest is the fact that it is a mimic of the neurotransmitter dopamine (Ernst 1967). Whilst opiate antagonists will prevent the emetic action of apomorphine, the relevance of dopaminergic mechanisms in the various opiate actions is unknown.

Miotic action

All the narcotic analgesics cause miosis. This is due to stimulation of the Edinger-Westphal nucleus of the occulomotor nerve centre. This is of clinical significance for three reasons. Firstly, in the common event of an opiate being used in anaesthetic premedication, the resultant miosis will interfere with pupil size being used as an index of depth of anaesthesia. Secondly, miosis accompanied by respiratory depression is a most useful symptom of opiate poisoning, easily distinguishable from the other major group of respiratory depressants, the barbiturates. Thirdly, miosis will still be present in narcotic addicts. Tolerance to the various actions of morphine can occur at different rates (p. 23). Little tolerance to this stimulant action of opiates occurs.

Other actions

Because of this confusing ability to excite and depress, and differences in this ratio between morphine analogues, the range of gross CNS effects is wide. *Sedation* leading to coma is the most likely outcome, indeed, so long as respiration is maintained, it is possible to produce surgical *anaesthesia* by intravenous infusion. On the other hand, *convulsions* can occur. These are cortical in nature, and because of differential rates at which tolerance can develop, may well be seen in dependent patients poisoned with a derivative possessing relatively high excitatory actions (e.g. pethidine). These convulsions can be prevented by phenytoin.

The opiates also stimulate the *release of the antidiuretic hormone*, causing a water antidiuresis.

Morphine has a negligible effect on cardiovascular control of clinical significance, though a peripheral action (p. 22) may become important. By and large, even during severe morphine poisoning, blood pressure is maintained and subsequent cardiovascular depression is secondary to respiratory depression and hypoxia.

Peripheral actions

Narcotic analgesics have two main actions in the periphery of clinical importance. They have actions on smooth muscle, and they can release histamine.

Smooth muscle

In man opiates increase the tone of smooth muscle. Clinically the most important consequence of this is on the smooth muscle of the gastrointestinal tract.

The constipative action of morphine and its derivatives is legendary. In man the mechanism of this action is an increase in tone of smooth muscle of the stomach, duodenum, small intestine and colon. There is also a decrease in propulsive movement in the small intestine and colon. In addition there is spasm of sphincters throughout the tract*.

The mechanism of this constipative action is unclear, though the possibilities have been summarized by Weinstock (1971).

It will be recalled that a peripheral action of morphine which has attracted much pharmacological interest is that on the isolated ileum of the guinea pig at which site morphine prevents the release of acetylcholine (p. 9). It would be convenient if one could use this *in vitro* mechanism to explain the constipative action *in vivo*. However, there is little evidence for this.

Amongst the other possible mechanisms is again the role of

---

* Spasm of the anal sphincter is the mechanism of that most unusual test for narcotic analgesic activity, the elevated Straub tail of the mouse.

morphine's subjective actions. Under the influence of the drug there is a decreased awareness of the necessity to defaecate.

Whilst all the opiates are capable of causing constipation, the ratio of constipative actions to others is not constant. There is a derivative of pethidine, diphenoxylate, which selectively shows the constipative actions of the narcotic analgesics in doses which have few other morphine-like effects (p. 63).

Opiates have other effects on smooth muscle. Of the greatest importance is their spasmogenic action on the sphincter of Oddi causing a marked increase in biliary tract pressure. Despite this the narcotic analgesics can still be of benefit in the treatment of pain from biliary colic, though exacerbation may occur.

Whilst opiates have parallel effects on other smooth muscle (e.g. ureter, urinary bladder, uterus and bronchi), these effects are seen only after very high doses and they are of negligible clinical significance.

Histamine release

Morphine and its derivatives cause a release of histamine. This effect is totally unrelated to interactions at the opiate receptor, it being only a consequence of the basic nature of the drug (see below). Histamine is bound in an inactive form with the acidic heparin. The introduction of a basic drug can displace histamine thus producing its unpleasant effects such as erythrema at the site of injection. This action is shared with other basic drugs such as atropine and d-tubocurarine.

Peripheral vasodilation, leading to orthostatic hypotension is one of the most apparent consequences of this histamine release, though it is of little clinical significance. It does, however, emphasize the relative lack of cardiovascular activity of these drugs since what little effect they have is due to an indirect action.

Bronchospasm is another manifestation of histamine release, and it may be dangerous in a patient with a history of allergic conditions. Certainly opiate derivatives should be used with great care in asthmatics.

Distribution of opiates in the body

The distribution of morphine and its derivatives has been reviewed by Way and Adler (1962), and by Lemberger and Rubin (1976).

The structure of morphine is given in Fig. 2.4 (page 19).

It is a weak base (pK_a 8·0) and, in common with most opiates, it is a tertiary amine. Note the two hydroxyl substituents (phenolic and alcoholic). Such substituents are polar and convey on the molecule a degree of water solubility unusual amongst alkaloids.

For this reason morphine is poorly absorbed across lipid membranes. The absorption of morphine across the gastrointestinal tract is clinically inadequate, and the drug does not penetrate the blood brain barrier with ease.

Fortunately some of morphine's derivatives are more lipid soluble than the parent compound (note the absence of polar substituents in the structure of pethidine, Fig. 3.4). Thus whilst morphine remains the type substance for parenteral administration, some of its derivatives are superior to it if the oral route is preferred.

The placental barrier is readily presented by opiate derivatives, hence the neonatal respiratory depression when the mother has received opiates during labour. It may also be noted that neonatal depression may be sufficiently marked to necessitate treatment even if the mother is showing no apparent opiate effects. The neonatal blood brain barrier is less selective than that of the adult, and opiates penetrate it with greater ease. In addition there are differences in the abilities of neonates and adults to biotransform opiates. The biotransformation of individual agents is described later (p. 42 *et seq.*).

Tolerance and physical dependence

Tolerance

Tolerance develops rapidly to some of morphine's actions. As an oversimplification, tolerance develops most to the depressant actions (respiratory depression, sedation, analgesia), but more slowly to excitatory actions. For instance, miosis is still apparent in narcotic addicts, and poisoning by pethidine in a pethidine addict may be manifest as convulsions.

The speed of tolerance development is considerable. Tolerance is apparent 4 hours after commencement of a morphine infusion in the experimental animal (Cox, Ginsburg & Osman 1968), and is likely to have occurred after 6–8 consecutive injections in man.

The mechanism of tolerance development is unclear, but it would seem to be unrelated to increased biotransformation (Mulé 1971). Tolerance presumably occurs at or beyond the level of receptor interaction. In the light of our recent knowledge of the existence of endogenous morphine-like compounds, many theories of tolerance development will benefit from re-examination.

Cross-tolerance occurs within members of the opiate group, though does not extend to other centrally acting drugs.

The extent to which tolerance develops is considerable. A narcotic addict may tolerate up to 500 times the clinical dose of morphine (i.e. 5 *gram*).

Physical dependence

Volumes have been written on this aspect of opiate pharmacology, and the interested reader might like to consult one of the comprehensive reviews (e.g. Jaffe 1975). The brevity of the following section is not intended to underestimate the gravity of the social problem that the opiates have caused, but to reflect on the relative unimportance of opiate dependence when the drugs are used in normal practice.

Physical dependence, though detectable, is unlikely to be significant following 2–3 days injections of morphine (as in postoperative pain), and is unimportant in terminal pain.

For the one occasion in which pure agonists are almost certain to induce severe physical dependence (chronic non-terminal pain), they are simply not used.

Bearing this in mind, some physicians are sometimes unnecessarily reluctant to use therapeutically effective doses of opiates in acute pain.

Whilst tolerance development is an early warning sign of dependence, tolerance may be unassociated with dependence.

It is virtually impossible to suggest a duration of treatment at the end of which withdrawal symptoms may be troublesome. This is because the frequency and quantity of injections, and duration of drug action all influence development of dependence. Nevertheless, it is apparent that, whilst withdrawal symptoms following termination of a course of clinical doses of opiates for periods of between a week and a fortnight will be detected, if the patient is not anticipating anything, the symptoms may pass by unnoticed.

The situation is different if withdrawal is precipitated by narcotic antagonists.

The symptoms of withdrawal are generally opposite to the original effects of morphine (e.g. diarrhoea, hyperventilation, mydriasis), the only exception being vomiting which is both an effect of morphine and a withdrawal symptom, though the mechanisms probably differ.

The symptoms will develop at about the time of the next scheduled dose and reach peak severity in 2–3 days. The symptoms will wear off during about one week.

Deaths have occurred during withdrawal. However, the number is relatively small (less than those deaths during barbiturate withdrawal?) and Glaser and Ball (1970) have doubted that death was due to withdrawal symptoms *per se* in any of a selected population.

It is not the intention of the foregoing to underestimate the problems of opiate dependence, but rather to balance the exaggerations that have been made in the past.

The problems of dependence on illicitly obtained opiates is a different matter, and leaves no room for complacency. The treatment of this form of dependence is a specialized topic, and is not covered in this monograph. In contrast, the treatment of 'therapeutic' addicts is not mentioned because it is so rare.

The narcotic antagonists

If Fig. 2.2 is reconsulted it is apparent that the pharmacology of narcotic antagonists must be considered from two angles.

Firstly, there is the pharmacology of an agent which possesses both agonist and antagonist activity and is given alone (e.g. pentazocine as an analgesic), and secondly, the pharmacology of the same drugs when given after a more selective agonist (e.g. naloxone reversal of morphine induced respiratory depression).

The pharmacology of nalorphine and pentazocine given alone

The observation that nalorphine possessed analgesic activity when given alone was one of those fortuitous accidents which so characterizes major pharmacological and therapeutic advances. Nalorphine had been used as a narcotic antagonist for some years and was the drug of choice to reverse morphine-induced respiratory depression. At this stage it was thought possible that a mixture of it and morphine might provide a more selective analgesic, the narcotic antagonist reducing the respiratory depression proportionately more than the analgesia.

With hindsight we now know that this approach is of no value (p. 17), but Lasagna and Beecher (1954) set out to investigate the analgesic and respiratory depressant actions of various permutations of doses of morphine and nalorphine. They also tested morphine and nalorphine alone, and it was to their surprise that they found nalorphine to be an analgesic.

It had already been established the year before that nalorphine did not cause morphine-like dependence since rather than substituting for morphine in a narcotic addict, it precipitated the withdrawal syndrome.

Nalorphine was tried as an analgesic in man. It was found to be relatively potent: 10 mg nalorphine had the same analgesic action as 10 mg morphine, though in contrast to morphine, elevation of dose caused no further increase in analgesic effect. In common with morphine it caused respiratory depression, nausea, miosis and constipation.

In contrast, its subjective effects were quite different. Nalorphine caused marked dysphoria, anxiety and, in a significant number of subjects, visual hallucinations, commonly of an unpleasant nature. The drug was abandoned as an analgesic.

Nevertheless once it had been established that a narcotic agonist also possessing antagonist activity could be an effective analgesic with negligible dependence potential, the search was on to find a nalorphine-like drug with less dysphoriant and hallucinogenic activity. The first product of this research was *pentazocine*, introduced in 1965, which is an effective analgesic by both parenteral and oral routes. Its subjective effects are more similar to nalorphine than morphine. Dysphoria is common, but with effective analgesic doses the incidence of hallucinations is slight.

Pentazocine possesses weak antagonist activity, which is insufficient to produce clinically useful antagonism of the pure agonists (cf. nalorphine). However, it can precipitate withdrawal in patients dependent upon pure agonists.

On the crucial question of dependence, it, in common with other partial agonists, does not cause morphine-like dependence. On the other hand, instances of a type of dependence have been reported. The characteristics of pentazocine dependence are that subjects initially experience euphoria after taking the drug (cf. above); dependence is rare; it takes a long time to develop; withdrawal symptoms (anxiety, sweating, lachrymation) are usually mild, pure agonists do not substitute for it and withdrawal can usually be tolerated without further medication.

Many of the early instances of pentazocine dependence were in members of the medical and paramedical professions. Availability has always been the major contribution to drug abuse.

Following the introduction of pentazocine onto the market as the first relatively potent non-addictive analgesic, its prescribing was widespread and often in the parenteral form (the oral preparation did not come onto the market till later). The observation of dependence promoted cynicism regarding the whole concept of non-addictive potent analgesics. However, this view tends to cloud the basic pharmacological fact that the dependence liability of pentazocine is less than that of weak agonists such as codeine and dextropropoxyphene. Nevertheless, whilst the proportion of patients who might become dependent is minute, such is the popularity of the drug that the numerical incidence of dependence may become significant (p. 58).

In view of the effectiveness of pentazocine, it is remarkable that no other antagonist analgesic has become clinically available until recently. The reason for this is that the vast majority of partial agonists, some of which are far more potent than pentazocine, are too hallucinogenic for clinical use.

Recently, a second narcotic antagonist analgesic has become available in the U.K.

Though there is currently an inadequate number of clinical trials to permit a full comparison, *buprenorphine* differs from pentazocine in the following ways.

It would seem to produce a greater maximum analgesic effect than pentazocine, and certainly has a longer duration of action. Buprenorphine does not seem to cause either euphoria or dysphoria. It causes more sedation than does pentazocine. Once the analgesic and respiratory depressant effects of buprenorphine are fully established it cannot be readily reversed by naloxone.

As with other opiates, buprenorphine can cause vomiting. The incidence of vomiting after buprenorphine may be greater than that commonly caused by the opiates and it may be persistent. Vomiting can be troublesome especially if the patient is ambulatory.

Antagonist actions

Naloxone is the only commercially available pure narcotic antagonist. In doses much higher than those necessary to antagonize a pure agonist, intravenous injection has no observable effects in control subjects.

Administration of doses between 0·5 and 1 mg will cause the most dramatic reversal of the depressant effects caused by a pure agonist. The most beneficial result of this is a reversal of respiratory depression and this will occur within a minute.

Figure 2.5 shows a spirometer recording of a patient during an intravenous injection of dextromoramide. Note both the short time it takes for respiration to cease after injection of the agonist and the impressive return to normal following the injection of the antagonist, in this case nalorphine.

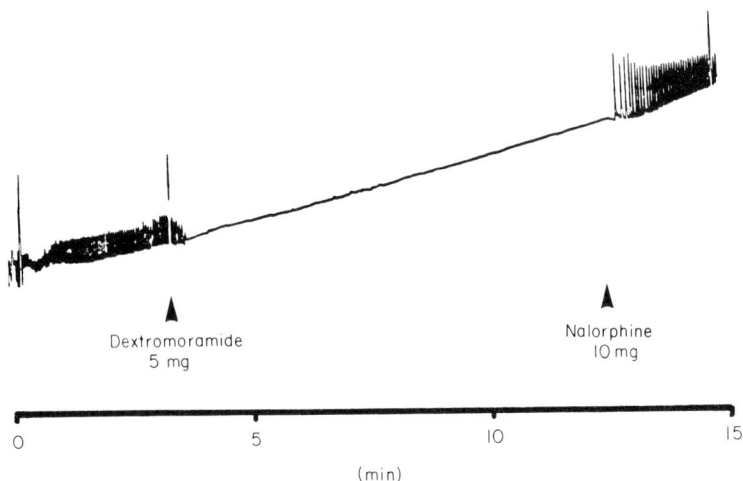

Fig. 2.5. A spirometer recording of a patient showing the cessation of breathing following intravenous injection of a typical narcotic agonist (dextromoramide), and the restoration of breathing following injection of nalorphine (From David & Delingé 1957, reproduced with permission, Masson S. A. Paris).

Naloxone is also an effective antagonist of the partial agonist pentazocine. Prior to the introduction of naloxone, non-specific respiratory stimulants (nikethamide, amphetamines) had to be used. Naloxone will also antagonize the dysphoric and hallucinogenic actions of the partial agonists, though higher doses may have to be used (10 mg).

In common with other drugs possessing narcotic antagonist activity, naloxone will precipitate the withdrawal syndrome. This will occur within minutes of injection, the withdrawal syndrome will be intense, but will wear off in a few hours (cf. spontaneous withdrawal).

It may also be noted that opiate antagonists may precipitate withdrawal in subjects in whom dependence would otherwise not be detectable clinically. Using narcotic antagonists the phenomenon of *acute dependence* has been identified following single injections of pure agonists.

Whilst naloxone remains an infallible treatment for opiate poisoning, a problem remains as to the treatment of opiate poisoning in the addict. The precipitation of severe withdrawal may be more hazardous than the respiratory depression. But if a narcotic antagonist is deemed necessary, small doses of naloxone should be given over a period of time, with great care.

It should also be remembered that death from opiate poisoning is due to respiratory depression, and that where facilities for artificial ventilation are available, this alone may be adequate treatment. The spectacular reversal of opiate depression coupled with potential precipitation of withdrawal may be dangerous to the patient and traumatic to the medical staff. Artificial ventilation may suffice.

Nalorphine and levallorphan differ from naloxone in that they are partial agonists. They may be relatively ineffective in reversing moderate respiratory depression and may even aggravate mild respiratory depression (a summation between two respiratory depressants). It would seem that severe respiratory depression and CO_2 accumulation is a prerequisite of reversal with these agents. They do not reverse pentazocine induced respiratory depression and both will aggravate non-opiate respiratory depression.

The molecular mechanisms of action of morphine and its derivatives

In retrospect, it is extraordinary that in 1970 few researchers insisted that a morphine-like compound must exist in brain. Even at that time all the pharmacological evidence necessary to suggest the existence of an endogenous morphine-like compound was available.

The narcotic analgesics illustrated more than any other drug group structural specificity in the central nervous system. The slightest change in structure leads to a dramatic change in pharmacological activity. For instance, while the laevo-rotatory isomer of morphine is the active pharmacological agent, the dextro-rotatory isomer lacks notable activity. The precise structure-activity relationships, and minimal chemical complement associated with opiate activity were clearly defined by this time (e.g. Janssen 1968). Such structural characteristics implied interaction with a receptor.

The gross structure of this receptor had been described as early as 1954 by Beckett and Casy, and subsequently a precise chemical structure was attributed to it (Loh, Cho, Wu & Way 1974).

The antagonism at this receptor between morphine and an antagonist had been proved to be competitive in nature both *in vivo* (Takemori, Kupferberg & Miller 1969), and *in vitro* (Kosterlitz & Watt 1968). In striking contrast to all other examples of competitive agonist–antagonist pairs, the interaction between morphine and naloxone occurred at a receptor for which there was no known physiological agonist.

All the above pointed to the existence of an endogenous morphine-like compound. Nevertheless, it was commonly believed that no such compound existed. Martin, one of the most eminent researchers and reviewers of the opiate analgesics argued in 1967 that no such compound existed, and the majority of researchers shared his scepticism. Even with hindsight, their scepticism was well-founded.

Firstly, whilst knowledge of chemical transmission in the central nervous system was still in its infancy, knowledge of the biochemical content of the brain was well known. No known compound seemed to match the minimal molecular complement of the opiates, and certainly none was known to possess morphine-like activity.

Secondly, were there to be an endogenous agent with morphine-like activity possessing a physiological function, it would follow that all species possessing such a compound would be physically dependent on it. Yet it is apparent that such individuals are not dependent in the same way as individuals can become dependent on morphine.

Thirdly, and by far the most important piece of evidence lay with naloxone. If an endogenous morphine-like compound existed in the brain and had physiological function, the administration of a pure antagonist like naloxone would antagonize it, and produce a pharmacological effect, in just the same way as the administration of the antagonists atropine, d-tubocurarine, propranolol and strychnine cause profound effects by antagonizing endogenous transmitters. Yet naloxone was then thought to be devoid of pharmacological activity when given alone.

Some felt, therefore, that no such endogenous compound existed. Perhaps at that time too little attention was paid to the only alternative explanation, that there existed in the human brain a receptor which was more clearly defined than any other, interaction with which caused the most profound pharmacological change, yet its sole responsibility was to accommodate a chemical constituent of the latex of the opium poppy.

During the sixties and seventies understanding of chemical transmission in the central nervous system expanded enormously with evidence of central chemical transmission effected by acetylcholine, noradrenaline, dopamine, 5-hydroxytryptamine, some amino acids and peptides. The concept of presynaptic receptors modulating transmitter release developed. During that time researchers turned their attention to interactions of narcotic analgesics with these systems, and many of these interactions were impressive.

No-one embarked on the theoretically simple exercise of preparing brain extracts, and determining whether they did or did not possess morphine-like activity.

In the early seventies, Kosterlitz and Hughes became convinced that an endogenous morphine-like compound existed. Wisely, brain extracts were tested on isolated tissues known to be sensitive to opiate analgesics (p. 10). Early in the project they reported that an extract from pig brain, when applied to the isolated mouse vas deferens, depressed contractions in the same way as did morphine, and the extract was antagonized by naloxone (Hughes 1975).

The simplicity of approach to this hitherto baffling problem is noteworthy.

It is now known that at least two groups of peptides possessing morphine-like activity exist in the brain—the enkephalins and the endorphins.

The enkephalins

In 1975 Hughes, Smith *et al.* reported the chemical structure of their enkephalins. The structures of the two closely related pentapeptides are shown in Fig. 2.6. They differ only in the terminal amino acid, and are individually known as met- and leu-enkephalin.

Their distribution in the brain and in the periphery has been outlined by Hughes, Kosterlitz and Smith (1977), and is summarized in Table 2.2. The distribution is similar to that of specific opiate binding sites.

They have been postively identified as being neuronal in origin, and evidence for their release has been established.

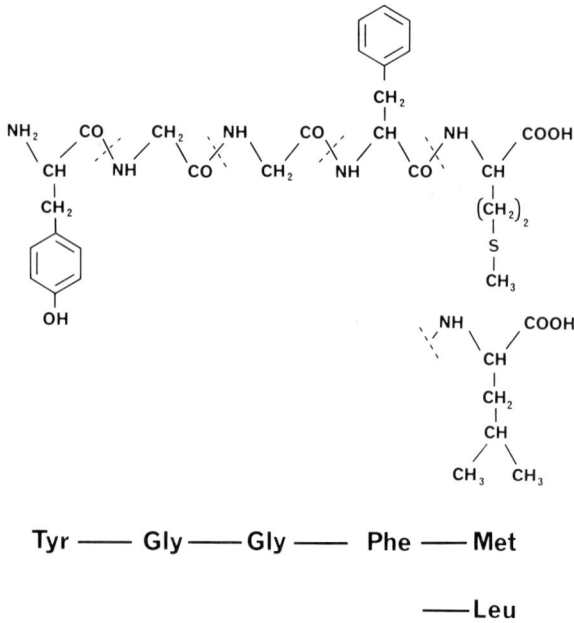

Fig. 2.6.

Table 2.2. The concentrations of met- and leu-enkephalin in various regions of rabbit brain. For further details (including the peripheral distribution of the enkephalins, and the distribution of endorphins) see Hughes, Kosterlitz and Smith (1977).

Brain region	Concentration (pmol/g)	
	Met-enkephalin	Leu-enkephalin
Striatum	681	209
Hypothalamus	575	100
Thalamus	162	38
Pons & medulla	145	50
Hippocampus	85	49
Cerebellum	52	< 10
Cortex	42	29

The endorphins

The term 'endorphin' is often used to describe fragments of the polypeptide β-lipotropin, and is sometimes used to describe *any* endogenous morphine-like compound.

β-lipotropin is a pituitary hormone consisting of 91 amino acids. Embedded within the molecule is the amino acid sequence of met-enkephalin (amino acid sequence 61–65).

Fragments possessing morphine-like activity include:

β-endorphin (C-fragment)	sequence 61–91
C'-fragment	61–87
α-endorphin	61–76
γ-endorphin	61–77

Their distribution differs from that of the enkephalins in that they are primarily pituitary in origin, though there are some located in neurones in the thalamus and hypothalamus.

The correlation between enkephalin and morphine structures

Structural correlations between the enkephalins and morphine have been made (Roques, Garbay-Jaureguiberry *et al.* 1976, Horn & Rodgers 1977).

Comparison of spatial models of the molecules shows some structural similarities which might escape the casual observer (Fig. 2.7).

The amino group of the benzene ring of the terminal tyrosine common to enkephalins and endorphins corresponds to that common to morphine derivatives.

The length of the ensuing amino acid sequence conveys some degree of stability to the molecule. Whilst enkephalin is rapidly broken down by peptidases, β-lipotropin is not.

Stability of synthetic enkephalin derivatives has been achieved by introducing different amino acids adjacent to the terminal tyrosine.

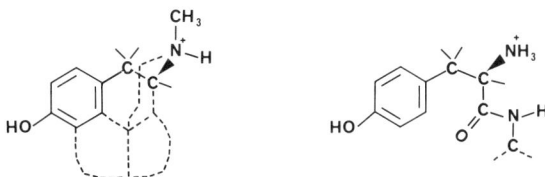

Fig. 2.7.

Pharmacological actions

The actions of the enkephalins and endorphins in animals are similar, the main differences being quantitative. β-endorphin is more potent an analgesic than is morphine, and has a comparable duration of action (Bradbury, Smyth *et al.* 1976). The enkephalins have a *very* short duration of action.

The peptides have analgesic activity in traditional animal tests following intraventricular injection. Synthetic peptide derivatives rendered stable are analgesic following parenteral and oral administration.

Met-enkephalin has been shown to depress respiration in the cat when applied to the ventricles (Florez & Mediavilla 1977).

Spontaneously firing neurones in the brain stem which are depressed by morphine analogues applied iontophoretically are also depressed by the peptides (Bradley, Gayton & Lambert 1977).

On the two peripheral models of guinea pig ileum and mouse vas deferens the peptides inhibit electrically induced contractions by preventing transmitter release—indeed it was on these peripheral models that the enkephalins were first characterized.

In all the above instances of some of the known agonist actions of endorphins and enkephalins, naloxone is an effective antagonist.

Predictably, though paradoxically, tolerance develops to the actions of the enkephalins, and there is cross tolerance with morphine (Van Ree, de Wied *et al.* 1976, Wei & Loh 1976, Waterfield, Hughes & Kosterlitz 1976).

Possible physiological roles for the enkephalins and endorphins

Most of the classical criteria which must be met before it can be claimed that a compound has transmitter function in the brain have now been satisfied (Fredericksen 1977).

1. Enkephalin is present in nerves.
2. There is a release mechanism.
3. The effect of locally applied peptide has the same effect as nerve stimulation.
4. There is a process for rapid inactivation.

The only criterion which is currently not satisfied is the mechanism of synthesis, though incorporation of labelled amino acids into enkephalin has been reported (Clouet & Ratner 1976).

Before considering evidence for a physiological role, it should be stressed that current thought is not that enkephalin has transmitter function in the same way as the major transmitters such as acetylcholine, dopamine and 5-hydroxytryptamine, but rather that it modulates the release of these other transmitters, just as it does in the periphery.

When considering the possibly physiological role of these peptides it is worth returning to the two paradoxes which contributed to the delay in the identification of endogenous morphine-like compounds (p. 29 *et seq.*).

If the peptides possess physiological responsibility:
1. Why are species that possess such compounds not dependent?
2. Why does naloxone have negligible pharmacological properties when given alone?

THE PROBLEM OF DEPENDENCE

It is clear that species (including man) which possess endorphins are not physically dependent *in the same way as a narcotic addict is dependent on morphine.*

There is no convincing explanation of this paradox. It could be argued that enkephalins have such a short duration of action that receptor activation is too brief to trigger off the biological change which is the mechanism of tolerance and physical dependence.

However, the endorphins, notably C-fragment, have long durations of action.

It could be argued that man *is* dependent insofar as an individual is dependent on any essential biochemical agent. Depletion (withdrawal) of essential central transmitters such as noradrenaline, dopamine and 5-hydroxytryptamine by reserpine causes physical changes.

Nevertheless, in traditional tests it has been shown that tolerance develops to the actions of the peptides, and they can induce physical dependence.

THE PARADOX OF NALOXONE

If the peptides possess a physiological role, the administration of their selective antagonist naloxone should produce pharmacological effects in the same way as the administration of other pure antagonists such as atropine and d-tubocurarine causes pharmacological

changes because of continuous physiological cholinergic transmission.

Before listing some 'fringe' actions of naloxone which might
imply a physiological role of enkephalins, two immediate explanations of the paradox should be mentioned.

Firstly, the enkephalins may not have any physiological role.
Secondly, naloxone may not be an effective antagonist of some of the
physiological actions of enkephalins.

These simple explanations should be considered, but at the
moment they are unconvincing.

SOME ACTIONS OF NALOXONE IN THE ABSENCE
OF EXOGENOUS OPIATES

Until recently it was generally accepted that naloxone had no pharmacological activity when given alone. The fringe actions of naloxone
listed below should not detract from this fact.

The following fringe actions of naloxone represent some of the
recent work, and between them they shed some light on 'enkephalinergic' transmission, and its physiological role.

1. *Analgesia caused by electrical stimulation of the brain*

It has long been known that electrical stimulation of various areas of
the brain will cause a specific antinociceptive effect (Mayer & Price
1976), and there has been some debate as to whether this is naloxone
sensitive. Akil, Mayer and Liebeskind (1976) demonstrated antagonism of analgesia caused by electrical stimulation of the periaque-
ductal grey matter of the rat by naloxone. Of significance is the fact
that the antagonism was only partial (40 per cent), and elevation of
the dose of naloxone did not cause greater antagonism.

2. *Pain threshold*

If endogenous peptides are involved in the establishment and maintenance of pain threshold, naloxone should be hyperalgesic. Published work is particularly confusing, the weight of evidence tending
towards a conclusion that naloxone has no effect on pain threshold.

Of interest is that Buchsbaum, Davis and Bunney (1977) have
demonstrated a hyperalgesic effect of naloxone only in those volun-

teers who were relatively resistant to pain. This raises interesting questions about the physiological basis of pain 'threshold' and pain 'tolerance', and the differential effects of drugs on these two possibly distinct parameters. After all, following injection of morphine in man, pain is perceived, but it does not matter so much (p. 15).

3. *Analgesia of acupuncture*

This is one of the clearest examples of an effect of naloxone in the absence of other drugs. It has been shown that naloxone can antagonize the analgesia of acupuncture in man (Sjölund & Eriksson 1976), and in animals (Pomeranz & Chiu 1976, Pomeranz 1977). It is reasonable to assume that peripheral stimulation of sensory nerve endings at sites determined empirically, causes central release of endogenous morphine-like compounds.

These findings may encourage scientific research into the phenomenon of acupuncture which has previously been ignored because it was not understood.

4. *Analgesia of stress*

It is well known that during stress, pain sensitivity alters. Analgesia can be produced in animals immediately following a period of stress.

Akil, Madden *et al.* (1976) induced analgesia in rats following a period of intermittent foot shock. This analgesia was partially antagonized by naloxone. Again it must be emphasized that the antagonism was not complete. Maximum analgesia was not significantly altered, but there was a significant shortening of the duration of analgesia.

It is significant that in the above example 'stress' was induced by a 'painful' stimulus, and the probability exists that pain as such can cause release of the endogenous analgesic.

Evidence for this has recently been obtained in man. Levine, Gordon *et al.* (1978) showed that naloxone enhanced postoperative dental pain. A more fascinating way of describing their findings is that naloxone will antagonize the analgesic action of placebo.

The above four examples of analgesia caused by mechanisms not involving drugs, but presumably involving the release of endogenous peptides represent some of the more important studies on the possible role of endorphins in pain sensitivity.

But it must be remarked that just because the most useful clinical action of morphine is analgesia, this does not mean that the most important physiological role of endorphins is on pain threshold.

All four examples have in common the circumstance of unusual physiological states (e.g. stress). The implication is that whilst endorphins may not play much part in the maintenance of pain threshold on a day-to-day basis, they may have a role in the modulation of threshold that *can* occur physiologically.

Of interest is that the peripheral site of action again provides a helpful model. Naloxone has negligible effect upon the transmurally stimulated guinea pig ileum (Kosterlitz & Watt 1968). Yet, following a period of tetanic stimulation Puig, Gascon *et al.* (1977) showed that the well known inhibitory phase which follows is antagonized by naloxone. A recording illustrating this is shown in Fig. 2.8.

Enkephalin is known to be present in the gastrointestinal tract (p. 31), and it is assumed that high frequency stimulation causes its release, and that it then inhibits, in this case, acetylcholine release. This action, like that of morphine, is presynaptic.

Whilst approaches to research may change in the future, naloxone has always been the key to understanding the physiological role of

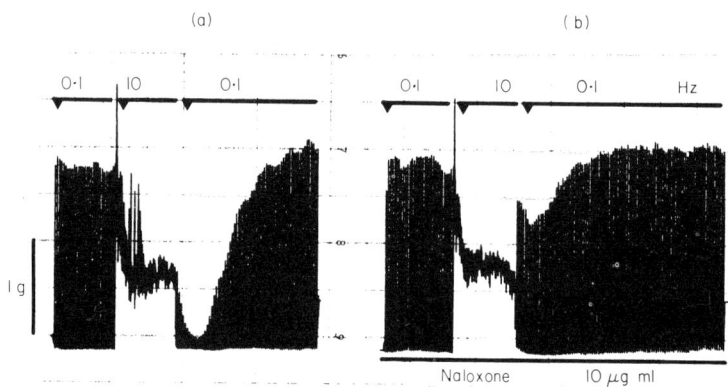

Fig. 2.8. Evidence for the *in vitro* release of enkephalin from the transmurally stimulated ileum of the guinea pig. (a) Electrical stimulation of the ileum at 0·1 Hz followed by a 5 min period of higher frequency stimulation (10 Hz). On returning to 0·1 Hz stimulation there is an initial inhibitory phase, and slow recovery to the original contraction height. (b) The same sequence of stimulation in the continuous presence of naloxone. Note the relative lack of a post-tetanic inhibitory phase, and the rapid recovery to original contractions.

enkephalins. Approaches may change with the availability of different pure opiate antagonists.

Bearing this in mind, two other actions of naloxone in the absence of exogenous opiates are of interest.

Firstly, the possibility exists that deficiencies in endorphin synthesis, release or metabolism may be related to a mental disorder.

Using the well established precedent of the use of hallucinogen antagonists in the treatment of schizophrenia, Gunne, Lindstrom and Terenius (1977) examined the effects of naloxone in schizophrenics. Naloxone is an effective antagonist of the highly potent hallucinogens amongst the partial opiate agonists (p. 27).

The cessation of auditory hallucinations which the authors reported was striking, though the duration of effect was longer than the accepted duration of action of naloxone.

Attempts to reproduce these results have been relatively unsuccessful, but it remains an attractive possibility that endorphin dysfunction may be correlated with a type of mental disorder. This possibility has recently been reviewed by Verebey, Volavka and Clouet (1978).

Secondly, naloxone has been reported to interfere with the actions of at least three drug groups whose primary effects are unlikely to be exerted at the opiate receptor.

Naloxone has been shown to antagonize the analgesic action of nitrous oxide in rodents (Berkowitz, Finck & Ngai 1977), to interfere with the behavioural effects of lysergic acid diethylamide in rats (Fertiziger & Fischer 1977), and to antagonize some actions of the centrally-acting sympathomimetics (Dettmar, Cowan & Walter in press, Little & Rees in press).

These three examples imply indirect involvement of endorphins in the mechanisms of action of some other drugs.

Reflections

What is the importance of these findings, and what developments can be anticipated in the next few years?

Firstly, there is the demonstration of a previously unknown biochemical system in the brain, interference with which has profound pharmacological consequences. The endogenous morphine-like compounds are unlikely to function as neurotransmitters in the same way as acetylcholine or dopamine. More likely they act as neuromodulators, modulating the release of the major transmitters in the

same way as morphine modulates transmitter release at some autonomic postganglionic nerve endings (p. 9 & 10). A specific demonstration of this presynaptic inhibition has been made by Jessell and
Iversen (1977). They postulate presynaptic inhibition of Substance P
release by enkephalinergic interneurones in brain stem and cord. It is
assumed that elsewhere in the brain enkephalin similarly modulates
transmitter release of other neurotransmitters.

Secondly, it is clear that an understanding of the physiological role
of endorphins will lead to an understanding of the mechanisms of
tolerance and physical dependence. This will not necessarily have any
effect upon the numerical problem of opiate dependence, nor upon
the success of its treatment. When a drug becomes available which
possesses potent analgesic activity and is devoid of all other actions,
thereby rendering traditional opiates clinically redundant, *Papaver
somniferum* will still grow, morphine will be extracted from it, from
which the synthesis of heroin is so simple.

Thirdly, and on a more optimistic note, there is the clinical possibility of opiates devoid of undesirable effects.

These may come from our new understanding of endogenous
morphine-like compounds, leading to the peptide analgesics, and
from the more mundane techniques of industrial screening of morphine derivatives.

Stable peptide analgesics are already known, and some show encouraging selectivity of action.

An early volunteer trial of such a compound produced surprising
and disappointing results (von Graffenried, del Pozo *et al.* 1978), but
by the time this monograph becomes available, many more studies
using different peptide derivatives will have been published, and it is
anticipated that more encouraging results will have been found.

But the goal of selectivity of drug action may be a result of pharmacological knowledge long known. Examples of relatively selective
morphine derivatives are already documented—dextromethorphan,
diphenoxylate and apomorphine.

Selectivity of action within a drug group often implies differences
in receptors.

Studies of the pharmacological actions of ketocyclazocine have
provided clear evidence of there being different opiate receptor popu-
lations. Ketocyclazocine has been shown to be a potent narcotic agonist devoid of antagonist activity, in contrast to its parent compound,
cyclazocine, which is pharmacologically similar to pentazocine. All

testing methods for dependence liability have proved negative (Villar-real & Seevers 1972, Swain & Seevers 1974). Such claims have of course been made in the past for many opiates, but there now exist many testing methods with good predictive ability for physical dependence in man.

Crucially, naloxone is a less effective antagonist of ketocylazocine than it is of morphine. This observation, coupled with many other studies have led to the suggestion of at least two types of opiate receptor (Hutchinson, Kosterlitz *et al.* 1975), or even three receptor types (Martin, Eades *et al.* 1976).

This may be the key. Over the last decades our understanding of chemical transmitters has led to the identification of three different receptors for acetylcholine, three for noradrenaline, and most recently, two for histamine. Identification of different receptors has led to drugs which mimic or antagonize selectively at each receptor providing more specific pharmacological agents.

However vital naloxone may have been in the elucidation of physiological roles for the endorphins, it may be that the endogenous compounds can act at receptors at which naloxone is an ineffective antagonist.

It is certain that in the central nervous system there is a range of opiate receptors, selective interactions with one of which will result in more selective pharmacological responses.

Chapter 3· Narocotic Analgesics and Antagonists
II. Individual agents and mixtures

Pure agonists

i. Controlled drugs. Class A.*

MORPHINE

Morphine is the standard narcotic analgesic with which other analgesics are compared. It is the most important alkaloid extracted from opium which is the dried milky exudate of the incized unripe seed capsule of the poppy plant *Papavera somniferum*.

In man, morphine is promptly absorbed after parenteral injection, but absorption by mouth is poor (Way & Adler 1962). Free morphine rapidly leaves the blood stream and is concentrated in parenchymatous tissue. Morphine does not accumulate and tissue levels are very low 24 hours after the last dose. The major pathway for metabolism of morphine is conjugation with glucuronic acid. Many narcotic analgesics are N-demethylated in man (e.g. pethidine, codeine and propoxyphene) and at least two hypotheses have been proposed implicating N-demethylation in the pharmacological activity of morphine and its surrogates. Beckett, Casy and Harper (1956) related N-demethylation to the analgesic action of narcotic analgesics and Axelrod (1956 a, b) related N-demethylation to the development of tolerance. Oxidation of morphine to pseudomorphine with consequent pharmacological implications has also been proposed. However, there is little evidence that N-demethylation is an important metabolic pathway for morphine (Way & Adler 1962) and the pseudomorphine hypothesis has received no support from experimental evidence (Krueger, Eddy & Sumwalt 1941). Some of the proposed metabolic pathways for morphine are shown in Fig. 3.1.

* See Misuse of Drugs Act, 1971.

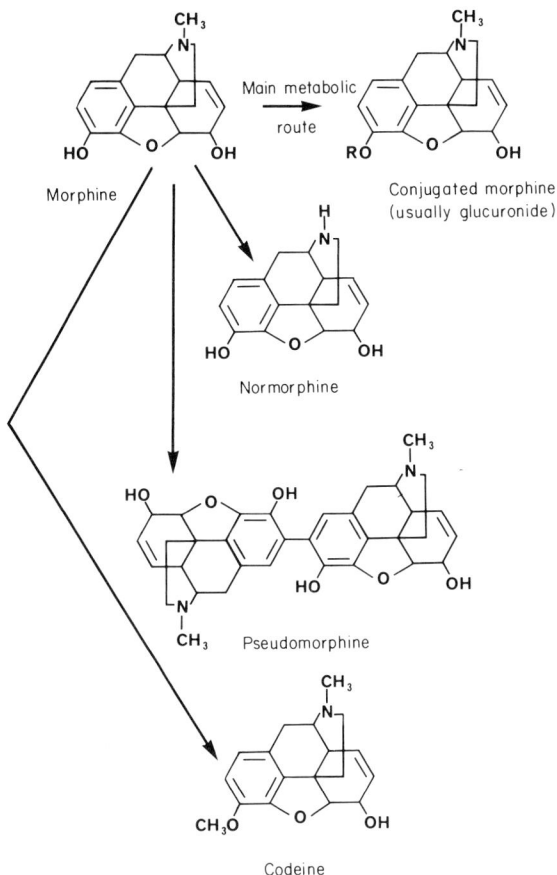

Fig. 3.1. Possible pathways of morphine metabolism.

Excretion of morphine is mainly in the urine and in man only about 5 per cent of the administered dose appears as unchanged drug. Some excretion occurs in faeces and bile and other fluids such as saliva, milk and perspiration play a minor role in morphine excretion (Way & Adler 1962).

There is no doubt that morphine is a potent and effective analgesic and whilst many newer analgesic agents have been introduced few, if any, are its clinical superior.

Morphine is usually given parenterally as its oral activity is low. However it is possible to obtain significant pain relief using the oral route of administration (Lasagna 1964). Increasing the dose of morphine increases analgesic activity, but unfortunately side effects are also increased. The usual parenteral dose is 10 to 15 mg per 70 kg man and this may be associated with significant respiratory depression (p. 17, Dripps & Comroe 1945). Other side effects of morphine include nausea, vomiting and constipation. The last named effect is utilized in some diarrhoea mixtures such as Kaolin and Morphine mixture B.N.F. Morphine may also cause spasm of smooth muscle and its use has been associated with a spasm of the bile duct giving rise to biliary colic. In man, morphine causes miosis, whilst in other species, for example the cat and monkey, it causes mydriasis.

The development of tolerance and physical dependence to morphine limits its clinical use. Furthermore, its abuse potential makes its use subject to stringent legal restrictions. Dependence and abuse of narcotic analgesics are discussed in greater detail elsewhere (p. 23).

DEXTROMORAMIDE

Dextromoramide is a high potency narcotic analgesic structurally related to methadone. 5 to 7·5 mg of dextromoramide are considered to be equipotent with 10 mg morphine for the relief of moderate to severe pain (Lasagna 1964). The drug is active by both oral and parenteral routes and Matts *et al.* (1964) found 10 mg dextromoramide to be equipotent with 100 mg pethidine for the oral relief of severe pain.

Most studies have found that dextromoramide produces more side effects than equianalgesic doses of morphine (Lasagna 1964) although Matts *et al.* (1964) suggested that dextromoramide exhibited slightly fewer side effects than either methadone or pethidine when given orally. In a study of the use of dextromoramide in obstetrical analgesia, Black (1966) was forced to discontinue the trial because of the unacceptably high incidence of side effects. These included respiratory depression, narcosis, nausea and vomiting and lethargy in the neonate. Black (1966) concluded that dextromoramide was neither useful nor safe for use in obstetrics and indeed it is not recommended for use in these circumstances (see Martindale's Extra Pharmacopoeia 1972).

There have been many reports on the dependence liability of dextromoramide and Seymour-Shove and Wilson (1967) reported two cases of dependence after dextromoramide had been used to treat mild pain of a temporary nature.

Dextromoramide appears to have no significant advantages over other narcotics, such as morphine.

DIPIPANONE

Dipipanone is a piperidino analogue of methadone. It is well absorbed from the gastrointestinal tract and may be administered by the oral route. It is metabolized in the liver and is excreted in both urine and faeces.

It is generally agreed that 25 mg of dipipanone is equivalent to 10 mg of morphine in terms of duration and intensity of analgesic action (Lasagna 1964). Whilst some workers have suggested that dipipanone is less respiratory depressant than equianalgesic doses of morphine, the consensus of opinion does not support this view and as with other narcotic analgesics side effects increase with increasing dose (Lasagna 1964).

However, unlike morphine, dipipanone has little hypnotic activity and when it is used for pre-delivery sedation, it is considered to be inferior to other narcotic analgesics such as pethidine (Johnstone 1958).

FENTANYL

Fentanyl, like phenoperidine, is related to pethidine although its duration of action is shorter than both pethidine and phenoperidine. Fentanyl is more extensively metabolized than phenoperidine, only 10 per cent being excreted unchanged in the urine.

Morrison *et al.* (1971) estimated that 0·2 mg of fentanyl was as effective as an analgesic for relief of post-operative pain as 10 mg of morphine, a finding which correlates well with the work of Finch and DeKornfeld (1967). However, the latter authors also observed that this dose of fentanyl was more respiratory depressant than 10 mg morphine and that fentanyl caused pain on injection. Furthermore, Downes, Kemp and Lambertsen (1967) observed that fentanyl caused a greater maximum depression of ventilation than an equianalgesic dose of pethidine, but that the depression was of shorter duration.

Whilst the duration of a single moderate dose of fentanyl is about 30 minutes, higher doses or repeat doses can produce respiratory depression lasting some hours. This may require the use of a narcotic antagonist.

Fentanyl is most frequently used in conjunction with droperidol for the technique of neuroleptanalgesia. There is some controversy as to whether droperidol increases the analgesic and respiratory depressant action of fentanyl in man (Fox *et al.* 1967, Kallos & Smith 1969,

Foldes *et al.* 1964). Certainly, the use of fentanyl and droperidol can result in post-operative respiratory depression (Morgan, Lumley & Gillies 1974).

HEROIN

Heroin, diacetylmorphine, is a semisynthetic derivative of morphine with potent analgesic activity.

Heroin is rapidly absorbed after parenteral injection, marked systemic effects being observed within two minutes of a subcutaneous injection. Oral absorption is erratic however, although generally effects are seen 20 to 30 minutes after ingestion (Way & Adler 1962).

Deacetylation of heroin occurs rapidly in the body yielding first monoacetylmorphine (MAM) and then morphine (Fig. 3.2). The

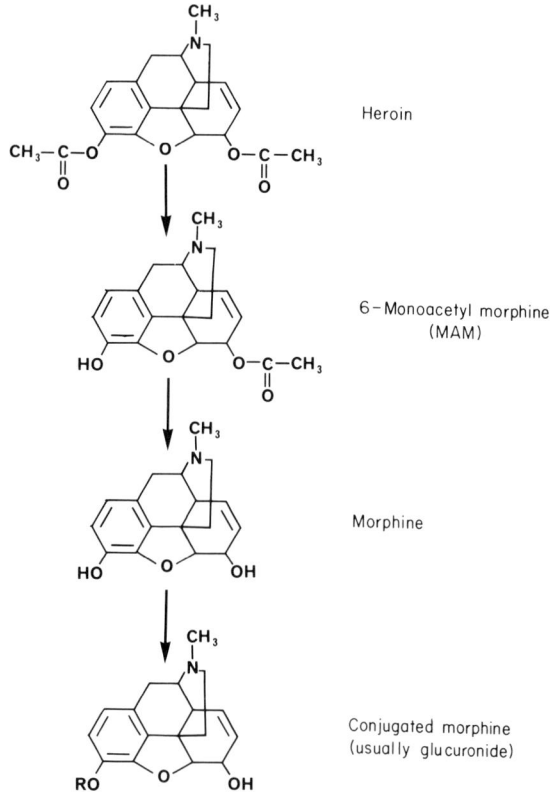

Fig. 3.2. Metabolic pathway of heroin.

morphine is then conjugated, probably with glucuronic acid. Many tissues are capable of deacetylating heroin, including brain, blood, liver and kidney (Way & Adler 1962). Indeed even in solution heroin readily deacetylates and thus heroin injection should always be freshly prepared (Davey & Murray 1969). After injection the initial conversion of heroin to MAM is so fast that very little of the pharmacological action of heroin can be attributed to the unchanged parent compound. Furthermore, it has been suggested that both heroin and MAM function mainly as carriers to facilitate the entry of morphine to its receptor sites in the central nervous system (Scrafani & Clouet 1971).

The major metabolite of heroin excreted in the urine is the glucuronide of morphine. There is no evidence that unchanged heroin is excreted in any significant amounts (Way & Adler 1962).

5 mg of heroin is considered to be equipotent with 10 mg of morphine with regard to intensity of analgesic action. However, the duration of heroin's action is shorter, about 2 hours. Whilst it is widely stated that heroin produces less respiratory depression than equianalgesic doses of morphine, controlled trials have been unable to distinguish between the respiratory depressant actions of the two drugs in both volunteers and patients (Lasagna 1964).

Other 'reported' differences between morphine and heroin have failed to be demonstrable in clinical trials. Lasagna *et al.* (1955) failed to find any convincing evidence that it was easier to acquire addiction to heroin than to morphine. However, heroin is widely abused throughout the world and in many countries is not clinically available.

Both Lasagna (1946) and Morrison *et al.* (1971) concluded that heroin and morphine were essentially similar in the quality of their actions.

However, heroin is still used by some authorities because of the clinical impressions that it causes more sedation and less nausea and vomiting than comparable doses of morphine.

LEVORPHANOL

Levorphanol is a synthetic analgesic of the morphinan series. The product obtained by synthesis is the racemate known as racemorphan, but the two isomers can be separated as the tartrates. The l-isomer, levorphanol (sometimes known as levorphan), has marked analgesic and respiratory depressant activity, but the d-isomer, dextrorphan, is virtually inactive in these respects (Benson, Stefko & Randall 1953).

Levorphanol and racemorphan are rapidly absorbed by both the parenteral and oral route. Traces of levorphanol may persist in the gastrointestinal tract for many hours, as the drug is actively secreted in the gastric juice (Way & Adler 1962). Metabolism is mainly by conjugation with glucuronic acid and the conjugate is excreted in the urine.

Levorphanol is more potent as an analgesic than morphine, 2 mg being equivalent to 10 mg of morphine given parenterally (Lasagna 1964). Although the oral potency of levorphanol is not as great as originally suggested, its oral parenteral potency ratio is better than morphine. In equianalgesic doses, levorphanol has at least the same dependence liability, respiratory depressant and spasmogenic properties as morphine. However, it does appear to have less sedative properties than other narcotic analgesics and it emerged as the best analgesic in a trial requiring analgesia with minimal depression of consciousness (Morrison *et al.* 1971).

METHADONE

Methadone is a completely synthetic narcotic analgesic whose chemical formula only remotely resembles morphine. However, its qualitative properties are similar to those of the natural alkaloid. The compound available commercially is the racemate, but most if not all of the analgesic activity resides in the l-isomer at clinical doses.

Methadone is well absorbed when given by subcutaneous injection or by the oral route. Methadone is strongly bound to tissue protein and, when administration is discontinued, low plasma levels of methadone are maintained by slow release from extravascular binding sites (Dole & Kreek 1973). This may account for the cumulative effects of repeat doses of methadone, the apparent slow development of tolerance and the prolonged suppression of heroin withdrawal syndrome by this drug.

Methadone is biotransformed in the liver. N-demethylation appears to be an important pathway and there is some evidence that this metabolite becomes an endocyclic compound (Beckett *et al.* 1968; Fig. 3.3). Less than 10 per cent methadone is excreted unchanged and excretion is mainly in the bile and urine.

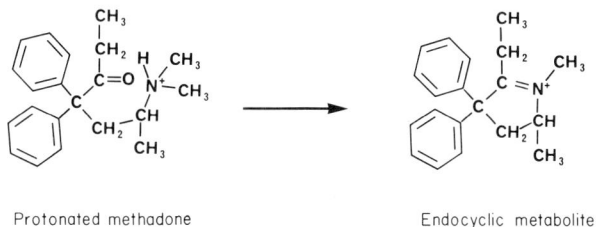

Protonated methadone   Endocyclic metabolite

Fig. 3.3. Possible metabolites of methadone (adapted from Beckett *et al.* 1968).

On a milligram basis, methadone has similar or slightly greater analgesic activity to morphine and like morphine the usual clinical dose is 10 mg. Whilst methadone is reputedly highly active by the oral route, clinical evidence confirming this is sparse (Lasagna 1964). In general equianalgesic doses of methadone have similar side effects to morphine although a single dose is less hypnotic. However, repeat doses are sedative and have a longer duration of action due to cumulative effects.

Methadone is also a potent cough suppressant but, since methadone is morphine-like in its dependence liability and cough suppressants are available with no dependence liability, its use as an antitussive has waned (Eddy *et al.* 1970).

Methadone is also used as maintenance therapy for heroin addicts.

OXYCODONE

Oxycodone, dihydroxycodeinone, has been recommended for pain relief as an alternative to morphine. The pectinate, which is usually given by the intramuscular route, has a duration of action about three times as long as morphine or pethidine (Brittain 1959). Well controlled clinical comparisons between oxycodone and other narcotic analgesics are few. In a double-blind study of 14 narcotic analgesics for the relief of postoperative pain, Morrison *et al.* (1971) concluded that the analgesic efficacy of 10 mg oxycodone was equivalent to that of 100 mg pethidine or 10 mg morphine.

It was originally thought that the dependence liability of oxycodone was less than that of morphine, however, Bloomquist (1963) demonstrated that its addiction liability was at least as bad as that of morphine.

Oxycodone has also been presented as a combination with aspirin, but Moertal *et al.* (1974) found that although this combination was superior to aspirin alone, it was not superior to aspirin codeine mixtures. Thus, in view of the greater addiction liability of oxycodone over codeine, there is little to recommend the mixture.

PETHIDINE

Pethidine, sometimes known as meperidine, is a synthetic narcotic analgesic, which, after morphine, is probably the most widely used potent analgesic.

Pethidine is well absorbed by all routes of administration although its action is less reliable when given by mouth (Lasagna 1964). After oral administration peak blood levels of pethidine are obtained in 1 to 2 hours. However, after intravenous injection blood levels fall rapidly for the first 2 hours and then more slowly. Pethidine crosses the placental barrier (Reddin 1966) and can be detected in the urine of infants born to mothers who have received the drug during labour. Recent studies suggest that pethidine accumulates in the fetus as the fetus has higher blood concentrations than the mother if the dose-delivery time exceeds 140 minutes (Caldwell *et al.* 1977). Furthermore these authors found that the half life of pethidine was only 2·8 hours in the mother but 22·7 hours in the neonate showing the relative inability of the infant to eliminate the drug.

Metabolism of pethidine occurs in the liver and N-demethylated derivatives account for one third of the administered dose. Hydrolysis occurs to both the parent compound, pethidine and to its N-demethylated derivative, norpethidine, producing pethidinic acid and norpethidinic acid respectively. Both these acids may be partially conjugated before excretion in the urine (Fig. 3.4). Very little pethidine is excreted unchanged (Way & Adler 1962).

Given parenterally, it has been estimated that 50 mg of pethidine produces lower peak analgesia and 100 mg produces higher peak analgesia than 10 mg morphine (Lasagna 1964). However, the duration of the action of pethidine is shorter than that of morphine, thus more frequent repeat injections are necessary for continuing pain relief. The respiratory depressant effects of therapeutic doses of pethidine are similar to those of morphine although pethidine may have less effect on respiratory rate, but more on tidal volume (Lasagna 1964). Some of the popularity of pethidine for use during labour

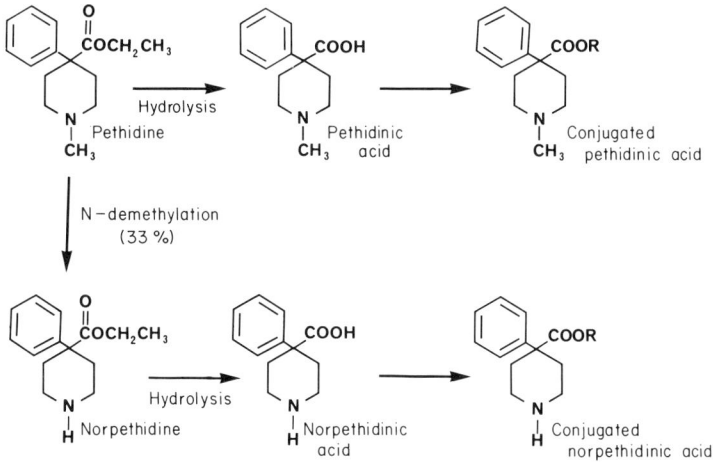

Fig. 3.4. Metabolic pathways of pethidine.

rested on reports that pethidine was less respiratory depressant in the neonate than other analgesic agents. However, Campbell *et al.* (1961) found morphine and pethidine to be equally respiratory depressant in the neonate.

Pethidine produces most of the typical narcotic analgesic side effects such as nausea, vomiting and sedation. There is no consistent evidence that pethidine produces less gastrointestinal effects such as constipation (Lasagna 1964), but its atropinic action should make it less likely than morphine to produce biliary colic.

Tolerance and physical dependence occur with pethidine, but the withdrawal syndrome is reputed to be milder with less autonomic effects and of shorter duration. Tolerance occurs more readily to the depressant actions of pethidine, than to the excitatory actions and thus repeated doses in addicts can give rise to hyperactive reflexes and convulsions. Reversal of large doses of pethidine with nalorphine may also precipitate convulsions. Work on monkeys suggests that the convulsant principle is the metabolite of pethidine, norpethidine (Deneau & Nakai 1961) and that convulsions can be expected in situations where the actions of norpethidine supersede the depressant actions of pethidine.

PHENAZOCINE

Phenazocine is a benzmorphan derivative with morphine-like analgesic activity. 3 mg phenazocine, by the parenteral route, has similar analgesic effects and side effects as 10 mg morphine. The respiratory depression obtained with phenazocine may be greater than that of equianalgesic doses of morphine (Lasagna 1964). Phenazocine is not generally thought to be highly effective by mouth (Beaver *et al.* 1968) although some authors have found it satisfactory (Economou *et al.* 1971). Phenazocine is effective when administered by the sublingual route (Economou *et al.* 1971).

Economou *et al.* (1971) also reported that the sedative action of phenazocine appeared to be less than that of pethidine and the opioids and that nausea and vomiting were less frequent. The duration of action of phenazocine is similar to that of morphine, however, the development of tolerance is slower and the abstinence syndrome due to phenazocine withdrawal is mild and prolonged. This suggests that phenazocine may have cumulative effects and slow excretion in man.

PHENOPERIDINE

Phenoperidine is a derivative of pethidine characterized by high potency, rapid onset of action, intensity of its peak effect and short duration of action. 50 per cent of the drug is excreted unchanged in the urine, but the remainder is metabolized to pethidine and pethidinic acid.

Phenoperidine is usually administered in conjunction with a neuroleptic drug for use in the technique of neuroleptanalgesia. There are few reports in the literature concerning the action of phenoperidine alone in man. Rollason and Sutherland (1963) found that the actions of phenoperidine (0·5 mg per stone) were unpredictable, some patients being comatose and others requiring supplementary analgesia. Certainly the analgesic effect was found to be of short duration (about one hour) but often accompanied by profound respiratory depression which might require reversal with a narcotic antagonist. However, even in the relatively high doses used by Rollason and Sutherland (1963) phenoperidine had few adverse effects upon the cardiovascular system.

The marked respiratory depressant effects of phenoperidine were confirmed by Jennett, Barker and Forrest (1968) who found that 1·5 mg phenoperidine (per 70 kg) caused a more prolonged rise in Pa CO_2 than either 10 mg morphine or 20 mg pentazocine.

Morrison *et al.* (1971) found 2 mg phenoperidine to be approximately equipotent to 10 mg morphine as an analgesic for the relief of post-operative pain. This potency ratio was considerably less than that which had been predicted from animal experiments.

ii. Controlled drugs. Class B.

CODEINE

Codeine, 3-methylmorphine, occurs in small concentrations in opium, but commercial supplies are obtained by chemical conversion of morphine.

The absorption of codeine is at least as good as that of morphine and may in some circumstances be better (Way & Adler 1962). There is some evidence that the decreased polarity of codeine furnished by the methyl substituent, favours its absorption by the oral route (page 23). Certainly codeine is two thirds as effective orally as it is parenterally, this being an unusually high oral-parenteral potency ratio for an opiate (Beaver 1966).

The action of codeine is terminated by metabolism in the liver mainly to inactive conjugates with glucuronic acid (Fig. 3.5). However, a small quantity of codeine, about 10 per cent, is O-demethylated to form morphine. There is evidence in some species that conversion to morphine contributes significantly to the actions of codeine (Way, 1968), however whether this is true in man is still open to debate. Codeine may also by N-demethylated to norcodeine (Way & Adler 1962).

Only 10 percent of the administered dose of codeine is excreted unchanged in the urine, the remainder being made up with the metabolites described above.

With the exception of aspirin, codeine is the most widely used oral analgesic. Numerous trials have illustrated the analgesic activity of 65 mg codeine when compared with placebo and the more sensitive trials have also shown the 32 mg dose to have significant activity. Whilst Lasagna (1964) observed that the analgesic activity of 60 mg codeine was almost as good as that of 10 mg morphine, increasing the dose of codeine did not improve activity markedly. Indeed, it is more usual to compare the activity of codeine with that of aspirin. Codeine has been variously quoted as having 5 and 10 times the potency of aspirin by the oral route (Beaver 1966).

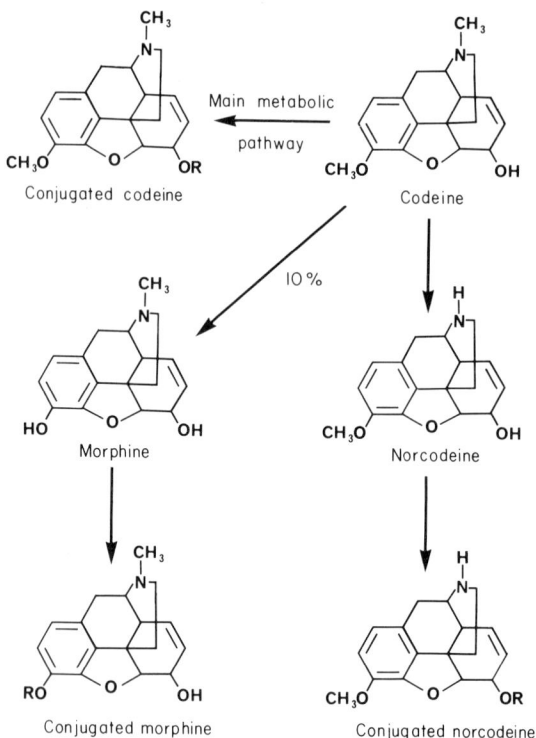

Fig. 3.5. Metabolic pathway of codeine.

However, codeine, like all narcotic analgesics, does depress respiration (Lasagna 1964). It also can produce nausea, vomiting, sedation, dizziness and constipation. These side effects become more frequent at higher dose levels. Furthermore, cases of primary codeine addiction have been reported (Beaver 1966) although it does not produce the psychic effects which most opiate addicts desire and is unacceptable to most addicts as a substitute for other opiates. Thus, the abuse potential of codeine is lower than most other narcotic analgesics and only mild legal restrictions are placed on its sale.

Codeine also possesses useful cough suppressant activity and is found in a number of linctuses for suppression of the unproductive cough. 30 to 60 mg of codeine generally induces significant cough suppression in man (Eddy *et al.* 1970).

The constipative effects of codeine have been utilized in some diarrhoea mixtures.

DIHYDROCODEINE

Dihydrocodeine differs from the structure of codeine in that it is saturated at the 7–8 double bond. It was originally introduced as an antitussive, but, like codeine, it also possesses significant analgesic activity.

Keats *et al.* (1957) considered that 60 mg dihydrocodeine was almost equipotent with 10 mg morphine in intensity of analgesic activity although Lasagna (1964) noted that the duration of dihydrocodeine's action was always shorter than that of morphine. There is evidence that doses of dihydrocodeine above 50 or 60 mg depress respiration. Indeed, Seed *et al.* (1958) concluded that dihydrocodeine possessed all the pharmacological properties of morphine in approximately the same relative potency.

However, at a dose of 30 mg dihydrocodeine has minimal side effects and may be equated with codeine for the relief of pain. It is active by both the oral and parenteral route.

Dihydrocodeine is also comparable to codeine for dependence liability (Eddy *et al.* 1970) and a few cases of dependence upon dihydrocodeine have been reported in the literature.

The antitussive action of dihydrocodeine is similar to that of the parent compound codeine and there is no evidence that it has any advantage over codeine for this purpose (Eddy *et al.* 1970).

PROPOXYPHENE

The analgesic activity of propoxyphene resides in the d-isomer of alpha-propoxyphene which is structurally related to methadone. The l-isomer is devoid of analgesic activity, but it has been used as an antitussive agent (Beaver 1966).

Propoxyphene is absorbed by both the oral and parenteral route, but like codeine, it is less effective by the oral route. N-demethylation of propoxyphene occurs in the liver and very little of the drug is excreted unchanged (Way & Adler 1962).

In a critical review of the analgesic trials concerning propoxyphene, Miller *et al.* (1970) concluded that propoxyphene is no more effective than aspirin or codeine and may even be inferior to these agents. Indeed, by the oral route, there is little evidence that the lower recommended dose, of 32 mg, has any analgesic activity at all.

Even in doses of 65 mg orally, Moertal *et al.* (1972) found propoxyphene to be indistinguishable from placebo, and significantly inferior to aspirin (650 mg) for the treatment of cancer pain. Combination of propoxyphene with aspirin was found to offer no analgesic advantage over aspirin alone (Moertal *et al.* 1974).

The side effects of propoxyphene include nausea, vomiting, sedation, dizziness and constipation. However, side effects are not a serious problem and it seems that propoxyphene is less likely to cause side effects than equal doses of codeine (Beaver 1966). In view of the inferiority of propoxyphene to codeine as an analgesic, however, it is debatable whether the comparison of effects obtained with equal doses of the two agents is meaningful.

Overdoses of propoxyphene have similar characteristics to other opiate overdoses, except that there is a greater incidence of convulsions. Overdoses have been successfully treated with naloxone (Kersh 1973).

Propoxyphene has less abuse potential than does codeine, but the characteristics of the abuse are similar to those of other narcotics (Beaver 1966).

ETHOHEPTAZINE

Ethoheptazine, ethyl-1-methyl-4-phenyl-1-azacycloheptane-4-carboxylate citrate, is a mild analgesic structurally related to pethidine. Whilst chronic administration has shown the analgesic activity of ethoheptazine to be significantly greater than placebo (Cass *et al.* 1958) this has not been the case in single dose or short term therapy trials (Beaver 1966, Moertal *et al.* 1972). The drug, however, is readily absorbed and peak blood levels occur 1 hour after oral ingestion.

When administered in recommended doses (75 to 150 mg), ethoheptazine does not seem to have significant side effects but toxic effects of high doses are manifest as central nervous system excitation. It has little dependence liability (Eddy *et al.* 1970) and in many countries it is free from the legal restraints placed upon the sale of codeine.

Commercially, ethoheptazine is usually available combined with other mild analgesics such as aspirin. However, there is little evidence that such combinations are more efficacious than aspirin alone (Moertal 1974, Beaver 1966). Indeed, the indications for the use of this compound would appear to be very small.

Pholcodine is a morpholinoethyl ether of morphine which is used almost solely as an antitussive agent. Its antitussive potency is 1·6 times that of codeine and, in contrast to codeine, it has little if any analgesic activity (Eddy *et al.* 1970). Whilst most of the clinical trials reported favourably on pholcodine and mentioned few side effects, they were not well controlled (Eddy *et al.* 1970). All that can be concluded is that pholcodine is an effective antitussive. Side effects which have been noted include nausea, constipation and drowsiness. It seems that pholcodine has less dependence liability than codeine, but since morphine can be synthesized from either drug legal restrictions exist upon their sale and manufacture.

Partial agonists

PENTAZOCINE

Pentazocine is the N-allyl equivalent of phenazocine and it was developed during attempts to obtain an effective narcotic antagonist from the benzmorphan group of compounds. Like nalorphine, pentazocine has both analgesic and antagonist properties, but the latter property is much weaker. Forrest *et al.* (1969) demonstrated that the analgesic activity of pentazocine resides mainly in the l-isomer, however, the commercially available compound is the racemate.

Pentazocine is effective when administered both orally and parenterally, but although absorption is reasonable by all routes, it is somewhat erratic in rate after oral and rectal administration. Peak blood levels are reached within 15 to 60 minutes after intramuscular injection but they may be delayed up to 3 hours after oral administration. Generally, the blood levels of pentazocine obtained correlate well with onset, duration and intensity of analgesic effect (Berkowitz 1971, Berkowitz *et al.* 1969).

Whatever its route of administration, pentazocine is extensively metabolized, only 2 to 12 per cent of the administered dose being excreted unchanged. Berkowitz (1971) found a correlation between incidence of side effects with pentazocine and degree of metabolism. Most side effects were seen in subjects who excreted the most free drug. The major route of excretion of free drug and metabolites (mainly conjugated pentazocine) is the kidney, only 2 per cent is excreted in the faeces.

The pharmacological properties, therapeutic efficacy and dependence liability of pentazocine has been extensively reviewed (Brogden, Speight & Avery 1973). The analgesic effectiveness of pentazocine for the relief of moderate to severe pain has been demonstrated in numerous controlled and uncontrolled trials. The peak analgesic activity of 30 mg pentazocine appears to be similar to that of 10 mg morphine when given by the intramuscular or subcutaneous route. However, since the effectiveness of pentazocine seems to decline more rapidly than does that of morphine, it is necessary to give 60 mg pentazocine to obtain the same total analgesia as that provided by 10 mg morphine (Beaver 1966). Orally, pentazocine has been found to be only one third as active as it is by the intramuscular route as far as intensity and duration of action are concerned (Beaver *et al.* 1968).

Like other potent narcotic analgesics, pentazocine depresses respiration. Although there is considerable argument as to the intensity of this action, a number of studies have shown that equianalgesic doses of morphine and pentazocine exhibit the same degree of respiratory depression (Keats & Telford 1964, Jennett *et al.* 1968). The respiratory depression caused by pentazocine cannot be antagonized by the narcotic analgesic antagonists such as nalorphine and levallorphan. However, it can be antagonized by the pure antagonist naloxone (page 28).

In contrast to morphine, which may cause hypotension and bradycardia, most investigators have found that pentazocine causes a slight increase in blood pressure and heart rate. This has been shown to be associated with increased circulating catecholamine levels (Tammisto *et al.* 1971).

Side effects with pentazocine are dose related and occur infrequently with recommended doses. Nausea, vomiting and dizziness are the most common, but the drug has also been reported to have psychotomimetic effects. Euphoria, mood alteration and sedation have also been reported.

Dependence and narcotic analgesic abuse are discussed more fully elsewhere (p. 2), however, it appears that pentazocine has low abuse potential and it is not controlled by narcotics regulations in many countries. Nevertheless, pentazocine is capable of being abused and both psychological and physical dependence have been reported

(Brogden *et al.* 1973). Indeed, in view of the easy availability of pentazocine, its abuse has become a significant clinical problem and reclassification of pentazocine as a controlled drug has been urged (King & Betts 1978).

Antagonists

NALORPHINE

Nalorphine, N-allylnormorphine, is a narcotic antagonist with marked analgesic activity. As an analgesic (Beecher & Lasagna 1955) and respiratory depressant (Foldes & Torda 1965), nalorphine is as effective as comparable doses of morphine. However, nalorphine's severe psychotomimetic activity makes it unsuitable for clinical use as an analgesic. The clinical use of nalorphine centres solely on its narcotic antagonist properties.

Nalorphine is rapidly absorbed after subcutaneous injection and the evidence suggests that it is more rapidly distributed and metabolized than is morphine (Way & Adler 1962). This probably accounts for its faster onset and shorter duration than morphine. Oral absorption of nalorphine is poor and the drug is not normally given by this route. Metabolism, mainly conjugation, occurs in the liver whilst nalorphine and its metabolites are excreted mainly in the urine.

Narcotic antagonists are used in the treatment of accidental narcotic-induced respiratory depression in a mother during labour and delivery, as well as for the prevention or treatment of the same in the infant. They are also used to treat narcotic overdoses, deliberate or accidental, and for the detection of narcotic analgesic addiction. All narcotic antagonists will reverse narcotic analgesic induced respiratory depression. However, if the depression is not narcotic analgesic induced, nalorphine, unlike naloxone, will cause further respiratory depression (Foldes 1973).

Nalorphine, like other narcotic antagonists, reverses both the analgesic and respiratory depressant actions of the opiates and thus administration before, or concurrently with, a narcotic analgesic, offers no advantages and will just lessen the activity of the analgesic. Nalorphine will not reverse the actions of other narcotic antagonist analgesics such as pentazocine. Thus, pentazocine overdoses cannot be treated with this agent.

Tolerance can occur to the agonist actions of nalorphine but since it does not support dependence of the morphine type (in fact, it precipitates withdrawal, cf. p. 26, it is viewed by addicts as an unpleasant drug and it does not produce the type of physical dependence that leads to drug seeking behaviour, hence nalorphine is considered to have little or no abuse potential (Martin 1967).

Many authors consider that there are few if any indications for the use of nalorphine when naloxone is available (Foldes 1973).

LEVALLORPHAN

Levallorphan is the N-allyl derivative of levorphanol a potent narcotic analgesic (see p. 47). Like other N-allyl derivatives it has narcotic antagonist activity. However, levallorphan produces less respiratory depression and fewer psychotomimetic side effects than nalorphine (Foldes, Swerdlow and Siker 1964).

The intrinsic analgesic activity of levallorphan, suggested by Martin (1967) was not confirmed in a recent volunteer study (Evans *et al.* 1974) although respiratory depression, a decrease in pupil diameter and psychotomimetic effects were observed. Although Foldes (1973) suggested that, in the absence of naloxone, levallorphan was the drug of choice for the treatment of narcotic depression, it is less popular than nalorphine in the U.K.

The duration of action of levallorphan is considerably shorter than that of the parent compound levorphanol and little is known about its absorption, distribution and metabolism save that its metabolism is more complicated than that of nalorphine (Way & Adler 1962).

NALOXONE

Naloxone, the N-allyl derivative of oxymorphone, is a narcotic antagonist. Unlike other antagonists, such as nalorphine and levallorphan, naloxone has no intrinsic analgesic or respiratory depressant actions of its own (Evans *et al*, 1974). Furthermore, it is the only antagonist, currently available commercially, which is capable of antagonizing the respiratory depressant actions of pentazocine.

Naloxone is usually administered parenterally as its oral activity is low. It acts within 1 to 2 minutes and its half life is about 20 minutes. Whilst intravenous doses of 0·4 mg naloxone have been shown to reverse the effects of quite high doses of narcotic analgesics, repeat injections are often required to prevent relapse into narcotic coma, particularly if a long acting narcotic has been administered. The short duration of the action of naloxone has been ascribed to rapid metabolism in the liver (Weinstein *et al.* 1973). However, the duration of naloxone's activity can be increased by administration of intravenous infusions or by intramuscular injections.

Even in massive accidental overdosage (20 mg to a 2·5 year old child—Rumack & Temple 1974) naloxone appears to be remarkably innocuous. Rare cases of nausea and vomiting have been reported, although no cause and effect relationship could be established. Similarly two cases of ventricular irritability have been reported in patients following cardiac surgery. However, animal experiments failed to demonstrate any increase in cardiac irritability induced by naloxone after morphine, although 2 out of 5 dogs used in this study exhibited cardiac irregularities coincidentally with the injection of naloxone (Michaelis *et al.* 1974).

Naloxone is indicated for the treatment of narcotic analgesic overdoses. Furthermore, its lack of intrinsic activity when given alone means that it can be used when the cause of the depression is uncertain. Naloxone, in contrast to nalorphine and levallorphan, will not add to the depressant effects of non narcotic drugs or pathological conditions. Successful use of naloxone for the treatment of non narcotic respiratory depression has been reported (diazepam—Bell 1975, barbiturates—Moss 1973), however, most investigators have found naloxone to be without effect in cases of non-narcotic poisoning (Evans *et al.* 1973).

In narcotic addicts naloxone will precipitate withdrawal and thus naloxone can be used to detect narcotic addiction (Blatchly 1973).

Naloxone is also used to terminate the action of therapeutically administered narcotic analgesics when the analgesia and concurrent respiratory depression is no longer desirable. The use of narcotic antagonists during labour and delivery has been reviewed by Foldes (1973) who concluded that naloxone was the agent of choice for the neonate. Subsequently many papers have appeared in the literature confirming the effectiveness of naloxone for the treatment of narcotic analgesic induced depression in the neonate (e.g. Clarke *et al.* 1975).

Recently, acute pulmonary oedema has been reported following naloxone reversal of high dose morphine anaesthesia (Flacke *et al.*

1977). The authors suggested that this was due to a massive sympathetic response to a sudden return of pain and they recommended that narcotic analgesic activity should be only partially reversed in such cases.

Derivatives with selectivity of action

APOMORPHINE

Apomorphine is obtained when the morphine molecule is treated with a strong mineral acid. Much of the analgesic activity is lost, but the compound retains the ability to stimulate the chemosensitive trigger zone and some other central excitatory and depressant effects.

Apomorphine is most frequently used by subcutaneous or intramuscular injection in the emergency treatment of noncorrosive poisoning where forceful emesis is considered advantageous (Done 1969). The action of apomorphine is not dependable when given by mouth. The usual dose of apomorphine is 0.1 mg kg^{-1} but it is not recommended that this should be repeated if emesis does not occur as higher doses of apomorphine suppress the activity of the vomiting centre.

Other uses of apomorphine include aversion therapy for chronic alcoholism (Moynihan 1965) and, since it is a dopamine agonist, as an alternative to 1-dopa in the treatment of parkinsonism (Braham *et al.* 1970).

Side effects of apomorphine treatment are persistent nausea, respiratory depression, sedation and hypnosis. It has been reported that the emetic actions of apomorphine can be antagonized by naloxone (Rausten & Ochs 1973).

DEXTROMETHORPHAN

Dextromethorphan, d-3-methoxy-N-methylmorphine, is related to levorphanol. Unlike its l-isomer, dextromethorphan has no analgesic activity in the usual analgesic tests, but it is a potent antitussive agent. Little is known concerning the fate of this compound, but animal experiments have suggested that its metabolic breakdown is more likely to be via N-demethylation than O-demethylation (Way & Adler 1962).

Although dextromethorphan has no narcotic analgesic activity,

Randall and Selitto (1958) have suggested that it may have some aspirin like anti-inflammatory action at least in the rat.

Dextromethorphan is approximately equipotent with codeine on a milligram basis as an antitussive (Eddy *et al.* 1970), but unlike codeine it rarely produces drowsiness or gastrointestinal disturbances. Whilst experiments show that the dependence liability of dextro-methorphan is either very low or negligible, some cases of dextro-methorphan abuse have been reported, although no withdrawal symptoms occurred after hospitalization (Eddy *et al.* 1970). Very high doses of dextromethorphan have been reported to depress respiration.

DIPHENOXYLATE

Diphenoxylate is a complex molecule linking the cyanide precursor of normethadone to norpethidine. It is used solely as a constipative agent in the treatment of diarrhoea. The compound is virtually insol-uble in aqueous solution and is only administered via the oral route. The drug is rapidly metabolized to diphenoxylic acid and currently no methods are available for its detection in blood or urine (Karim, Ranney, Evensen & Clark 1972).

The commercially available preparation 'Lomotil' also contains a sub-therapeutic dose of atropine with the aim of preventing excessive self medication. Barowsky and Schwartz (1962) found 2·5 mg of diphenoxylate in this combination to be as effective as 4 ml of Tinct. Camph. Co. for the treatment of diarrhoea.

In therapeutic doses diphenoxylate produces no morphine-like effects, but overdoses show typical narcotic analgesic symptoms. These overdoses are best treated with naloxone (Rumack & Temple 1974).

Chronic administration of diphenoxylate can lead to a morphine like physical dependence, but its insolubility precludes parenteral abuse (Fraser & Isbell 1961).

Drug mixtures incorporating narcotic analgesics

In the early part of this century it was rare for drugs to be prescribed in any form except as fixed dose combinations with other agents. However, the introduction of more potent and more selective agents, and a clearer understanding of the pharmacology of drugs and their interactions with each other, has resulted in a swing of opinion against fixed dose mixtures.

It is now considered that it is necessary to adjust the dose of each drug to the particular needs of the patient, in order to obtain maximum benefit from combined medication with minimum side effects. Furthermore, it may be advisable to stagger the timing of administration of the individual drugs, particularly if the duration of action of each drug is different. If toxicity or adverse reactions occur to a drug mixture it may be difficult to ascertain the causative agent and the management of such overdoses is complex. This is illustrated by the problems involved in the management of overdoses of 'Lomotil', an effective and useful agent for the treatment of diarrhoea. 'Lomotil' contains diphenoxylate, a compound related to morphine, and atropine as a deterrent to excessive self medication. Children are particularly susceptible to overdoses of this preparation and several cases of overdose have been reported in the literature. The initial signs of intoxication are usually typical of atropine poisoning, but these symptoms may subside and the patient be discharged from care, before the appearance of opiate type toxicity involving respiratory depression and coma.

Despite the above drawbacks to the use of fixed dose mixtures, there are a few advantages. If multiple drug therapy is required, the patient is more likely to take medication as directed if the drugs are combined in a single package. Occasionally, a drug does give more satisfactory results when combined with another. The side effects which occur after a combination of aspirin and codeine are considerably less than those obtained with equally analgesic doses of codeine or aspirin alone (Moertal *et al.* 1974).

COMBINATIONS WITH PHENOTHIAZINES

The rationale for this combination is to add the sedative and antiemetic effects of the phenothiazines to the analgesic actions of the narcotic analgesics. The popularity of such a mixture is shown by the marketing, in a single ampoule, of a mixture of pethidine and promethazine ('Pamergan'). 'Pamergan' is available in a number of dose combinations and may also contain atropine or scopolamine. It is recommended for use as pre-anaesthetic medication, for obstetrical analgesia and for the treatment of severe pain.

There is some disagreement in the literature concerning the effects of promethazine on the analgesic actions of pethidine. Peña (1965) suggested that the analgesic action of pethidine was enhanced, but Moore and Dundee (1961), in a study of experimental pain, found that 50 mg of promethazine inhibited the analgesic action of 100 mg of pethidine. These authors suggested that a lower dose of promethazine might produce the desired anti-emetic effect and sedation without undue reduction of pethidine's analgesia. Indeed one of the 'Pamergan' preparations contains only 25 mg promethazine ('Pamergan' AP100/25).

Thus, provided the physician requires to give a fixed dose mixture of pethidine and promethazine, 'Pamergan' is more economical on syringes, needles and the number of injections given to the patient. However, if repeat doses are required it should be noted that the duration of action of promethazine exceeds that of pethidine by at least an hour.

COMBINATIONS WITH BUTYROPHENONES

Combinations of this nature, notably fentanyl and droperidol, are used for the anaesthetic technique of neuroleptanalgesia and as anaesthetic premedication. The combination of drugs produces a state of analgesia associated with quiescence and indifference to environmental stimuli. Many anaesthetists prefer to administer each drug separately, but the mixture is available in a single ampoule containing 0·1 mg fentanyl and 5 mg droperidol in 2 ml ('Thalamonal').

Induction of anaesthesia with the mixture is slow as the peak effects of the drugs are not seen until 3 to 5 minutes after injection. There may be mild to moderate hypotension and the respiratory depression requires that respiration should be assisted (Dunbar *et al.* 1967). A few simple procedures are possible with fentanyl and droperidol alone but nitrous oxide must be added for full surgical anaesthesia. The major advantage of the technique is that analgesia extends into the post operative period. The incidence of post-operative vomiting is low and the cardiovascular stability observed in most cases gives neuroleptanalgesia (with nitrous oxide) some advantage over other anaesthetic techniques even in 'poor risk' patients (Morgan, Lumley & Gillies 1974).

A major drawback of the combination is that the durations of action of the two components differ markedly, the action of droperidol being much longer than that of fentanyl. Indeed, occasionally, central actions of droperidol such as extra-pyramidal disturbances or sedation may persist for up to 48 hours. Thus early discharge patients should be warned not to drive or operate machinery even on the day following administration.

COMBINATIONS WITH ANTIPYRETIC ANALGESICS

Examination of any current list of medical specialities will show that over 40 per cent of the oral preparations marketed for pain relief are fixed dose combinations involving an opiate with an antipyretic analgesic. The cynic might suggest that this was due to successful marketing policies, however there is some evidence that the two classes of drug may act synergistically to produce a more satisfactory degree of pain relief.

Recently Moertal *et al.* (1974) have confirmed that a combination of codeine and aspirin has significantly more analgesic activity than either drug separately. It is true that similar degrees of analgesia could be obtained by increased doses of codeine alone, but this would result in a vastly increased incidence of side effects. Moertal *et al.* (1974) also found that oxycodone with aspirin, and pentazocine with aspirin were as effective as analgesics as codeine with aspirin. However, since oxycodone has considerable abuse potential and pentazocine is expensive, codeine with aspirin would seem to be the combination of choice. It is interesting that the same authors were unable to detect any advantage of either ethoheptazine with aspirin or propoxyphene with aspirin over aspirin alone.

COMBINATIONS WITH NARCOTIC ANTAGONISTS

In the early 1950's some investigators postulated the combinations of narcotic analgesics and narcotic antagonists might counteract the undesirable actions of narcotic analgesics such as respiratory depression, sedation and addiction, whilst retaining the desirable analgesic activity. In subsequent years a number of reports appeared in the literature either supporting or denying this postulate.

Several of these conflicting reports were reviewed by Telford and Keats (1961) who found that the main problem in interpretation of results involved the relatively high precision available for estimating respiratory parameters coupled with very insensitive tests for analgesic activity. One paper claimed to show that levallorphan did not reduce the analgesic activity of pethidine, although their analgesic testing method was unable to detect the effects of doubling the dose of pethidine. Telford and Keats (1961) concluded that there was no evidence that the combination of a narcotic analgesic with a narcotic antagonist could reduce the respiratory depressant effect of the analgesic without affecting analgesia.

Nevertheless a mixture of pethidine and levallorphan is still marketed ('Pethilorphan') and the makers claim that in the doses used (Pethidine:levallorphan = 100:1·25) the respiratory depressant effect of pethidine is inhibited whilst the analgesia is unaffected. However, Morrison, Loan and Dundee (1971) found that the addition of levallorphan to pethidine, even in the proportion found in 'Pethilorphan', reduced the analgesic activity of the latter and concluded that the mixture had little to commend it in clinical practice.

COMBINATIONS WITH BARBITURATES

There are several of these combinations of which 'Sonalgin' is typical and contains butobarbitone 60 mg, codeine phosphate 10 mg and phenacetin 225 mg in a single tablet. It is recommended for use in insomnia due to pain, or for diurnal sedation.

The only advantage of this type of mixture is that the patient is more likely to take the medication as directed by the physician. This assumes however, that the physician has decided that the patient requires these three drugs in the doses provided in the tablet. The side effects of 'Sonalgin' are the sum of the side effects of the individual agents, the most important being the summation of the respiratory and cardiovascular depression produced by codeine and the barbiturates.

The barbiturates are considered to be antanalgesic (Dundee 1960). Thus it is theoretically possible that barbiturates might reduce the analgesic actions of codeine and phenacetin. Certainly, Moertal *et al.* (1974) found that the addition of pentobarbitone to aspirin tended to reduce the analgesic action of the latter, but not to a statistically significant degree.

A final point about combinations with barbiturates is that there has been a swing of opinion against the routine use of barbiturates as hypnotics or sedatives. The barbiturates have considerable abuse potential and habituation to the barbiturates is relatively common. Furthermore, cases of insomnia can often be treated by the establishment of a regular sleep routine without recourse to drugs. Even if drugs are used, the more selective action of the benzodiazepines are often considered preferable to the general depression produced by the barbiturates (Harvey 1975). In view of the doubts about the usefulness of the barbiturates themselves the use of barbiturates in fixed dose combinations with other drugs cannot be recommended.

COMBINATIONS WITH NON-SPECIFIC RESPIRATORY STIMULANTS

The ideal in analgesic therapy is to obtain complete pain relief without unwanted side effects. Whilst the opiates are the most potent and powerful analgesics known they also depress respiration and cause narcosis. A number of combinations of narcotic analgesics with respiratory stimulant drugs have been marketed over the years with the aim of abolishing opiate-induced respiratory depression whilst maintaining analgesic activity. The concept of this combination of drugs is attractive, but the problem is that there is no truly selective respiratory stimulant.

Mixtures of morphine and amphetamine have been tried, but they have not been found to be therapeutically useful, principally because of the cardiovascular side effects of amphetamine.

A combination of morphine with tetrahydroaminacrine ('Mortha') achieved limited popularity in the 1960's for the treatment of intractable pain and severe post-operative pain. Simpson *et al.* (1962) demonstrated that this combination of drugs had significantly less hypnotic activity than morphine alone and thus that the mixture would be particularly useful when it was necessary for the patient to be alert and co-operative. However, the lack of narcosis made the mixture unsuitable for pre-anaesthetic medication (Clarke & Dundee 1965). Tetrahydroaminacrine also has anticholinesterase activity and can prolong the action of suxamethonium or reverse the actions of tubocurarine. Whether this is an advantage or a disadvantage to the use of 'Mortha' during anaesthesia depends upon the end result required. Clarke and Dundee (1965) found that morphine and tetrahydroaminacrine enhanced post operative muscle pains after suxamethonium, but not all workers agreed with this finding (e.g. Thomas 1964). Similarly Clarke and Dundee (1965) found the incidence of vomiting higher on the mixture than on morphine alone, a finding at variance with some other studies (Stone, Moon & Shaw 1961).

Nevertheless, the general distrust of 'respiratory stimulants' and the swing of opinion against fixed dose combinations has resulted in the withdrawal of this particular combination from the market.

COMBINATION WITH OTHER OPIUM ALKALOIDS

Natural opium contains 25 per cent by weight of alkaloids. Morphine accounts for 40 per cent of these alkaloids and the remainder is made up of at least twenty other alkaloids, the most important being codeine, thebaine, noscapine and papaverine. The analgesic action of opium is due almost solely to the morphine which it contains. Opium is less rapidly absorbed than morphine and the presence of the smooth muscle relaxants papaverine and noscapine makes opium more constipating than morphine. Thus opium is used in a number of mixtures intended to treat diarrhoeas and colic, e.g. chalk powder with opium. Camphorated opium tincture (paregoric) delightfully described by Jaffe and Martin (1975) as a 'needlessly complex therapeutic survival of a former day', is also used to treat diarrhoeas and it is often combined with expectorants for the treatment of coughs. Adequate evaluation of many of these traditional cough remedies has probably never been carried out.

Papaveretum is an opium concentrate standardized to contain 50 per cent morphine. It is frequently used for anaesthetic premedication as papaveretum is reputed to have fewer side effects than morphine. However, a number of studies have found the action of 20 mg papaveretum to be indistinguishable from that of 10 mg morphine (Morrison, Loan and Dundee 1971). Administered parenterally, it is unlikely that papaveretum contains enough papaverine to have significant smooth muscle relaxant activity.

Chapter 4· Antipyretic Analgesics
I. Mechanism of action and general pharmacology

Historical development

The search for synthetic antipyretic agents was prompted by the high price of cinchona bark towards the end of the nineteenth century. Although the active principle of cinchona bark, quinine, was isolated in 1920, its synthesis is so complex and costly that, even today, quinine is obtained solely from natural sources.

Many compounds with analgesic, antipyretic and anti-inflammatory actions were introduced into medicine around the turn of the century, but they all lacked the antimalarial activity of quinine. The most important and lasting drugs to be developed during this period were the salicylates. The use of salicylates as antipyretic and analgesic agents was known in ancient time. Indeed the now discarded drug *Salicis cortex*, the bark of various kinds of willow, was once considered to be a rival of cinchona bark. The willow bark yields a bitter glycoside, salicin, which liberates glucose and salicyl alcohol on hydrolysis.

Salicin was used by Piria to prepare salicylic acid in 1853 and the first wholly synthetic salicylic acid became available in 1874. Within the next two years, Buss, and Stricker and MacLagen reported independently the successful use of sodium salicylate in the management of rheumatic fever.

Whilst acetylsalicylic acid was first prepared in the same year as salicylic acid, it was not used clinically until 1899, when Wohlgement and Dreser used it in the treatment of rheumatic diseases.

A more transitory popularity was achieved by acetanilid, which was introduced in 1886 by Cahn and Hepp. The compound was excessively toxic, but it lead to the development of similar drugs with less general toxicity whilst retaining acetanilid's useful properties. Phenacetin was the most satisfactory agent of those studied and it was used clinically soon after the introduction of acetanilid. A little later, in 1893, paracetamol was first used, but it did not gain popularity until 1949, when it was found to be the active metabolite of both phenacetin and acetanilid. Since this time a number of other antipyretic analgesics have been marketed and those which have achieved widespread use are discussed in Chapter 5. One of the most recent additions is diflunisal which has a pharmacological profile similar to aspirin, but has a longer duration of action and has less effect on blood platelets (Willoughby, Wright & Turner 1977).

Analgesic activity

The antipyretic analgesics have been found to be most useful for the treatment of headache, rheumatic and muscular pain, arthritic pain and pain arising from integumental structures. They are not effective for the treatment of acute pain of visceral origin.

The limited spectrum of the analgesic activity of these compounds may be due to a low ceiling effect and the differing intensities of the various types of pain. It has been suggested that the antipyretic analgesics only act on pain associated with inflammation and oedema. Certainly the antipyretic analgesics show inconsistent activity in analgesic tests utilizing non-inflammatory pain (Randall 1963) and many of the agents reduce inflammation in both the clinical and experimental situation (Beaver 1965). However, both phenacetin and paracetamol are effective analgesics which possess negligible anti-inflammatory activity. Furthermore, phenylbutazone is a potent anti-inflammatory agent with weak analgesic activity.

In 1959 Winder suggested that the mild analgesics owed their activity to a combination of weak central antinociceptive activity and an adjunctive property, perhaps an action on pre-inflammatory processes. Although the existence of a central component in the analgesic action of salicylate has been demonstrated in the rat (Dubas & Parker 1971), the importance of a peripheral action was demonstrated by cross perfusion studies in dogs (Smith & Smith 1966). It was shown that the response to the application of a noxious stimulus to the spleen, for example, an injection of bradykinin, could be inhibited by the addition of aspirin-like drugs to the circulation perfusing the spleen, but not by addition to the circulation perfusing the brain. The opposite results were obtained with the narcotic analgesics.

There is now considerable evidence to support the view that aspirin-like drugs block the production and/or release of an endogenous pain substance at the site of the noxious stimulus. The candidature of a number of substances has been examined in relationship to the actions of the antipyretic analgesics including histamine, 5-hydroxytryptamine, kinins and enzymes (Collier 1969). However, since the discovery that aspirin inhibits the synthesis of prostaglandins (Vane 1971, Smith & Willis 1971) attention has been focused on inhibition of prostaglandin synthesis as a mechanism of analgesic activity as well as anti-inflammatory and antipyretic activity.

The prostaglandins E_1 and E_2 (PGE_1 and PGE_2) are powerful irritants in the mouse (Collier & Schneider 1972) and produce headaches and pain on injection in man (Ferreira & Vane 1974). Furthermore, they appear to sensitize 'Pain' receptors to other noxious substances such as histamine and bradykinin (Ferreira, Moncado & Vane 1971).

Ferreira *et al.* (1971) suggested that the analgesia produced by aspirin-like drugs *could* be explained by the removal of the facilitation produced by endogenously released prostaglandins, which normally lead to hyperalgesia to mechanical or chemical stimulation. Such an action would explain the weak analgesic activity of aspirin-like drugs.

Anti-inflammatory activity

Many of the antipyretic analgesics possess marked anti-inflammatory activity, the exceptions being the para-aminophenol derivatives phenacetin and paracetamol (Adams 1960). Over the years a number of hypotheses have been advanced to explain anti-inflammatory activity including interference with oxidative phosphorylation, displacement of an endogenous anti-inflammatory peptide, interference with migrating leucocytes and inhibition of the generation of lipoperoxides (Ferreira & Vane 1974).

However, the discovery that aspirin-like drugs inhibit prostaglandin synthesis (Vane 1971, Smith & Willis 1971) prompted studies on a possible role of prostaglandins in inflammation and inhibition of prostaglandin synthesis as a mechanism of anti-inflammatory activity.

Flower *et al.* (1972) noted that the rank order of aspirin-like drugs against spleen prostaglandin synthetase was similar to that for inhibition of carrageenin rat paw oedema. Furthermore, optical isomers of anti-inflammatory agents which have little intrinsic anti-inflammatory properties also have low prostaglandin synthetase inhibitory activity.

A number of mediators have a role in inflammation. For example, in rat paw oedema induced by carrageenin, Di Rosa *et al.* (1971 a, b) found that the first phase of the response appeared to involve histamine and 5-hydroxytryptamine, a second phase involved bradykinin and thereafter prostaglandins were released. This last 'prostaglandin phase' was most susceptible to aspirin. Evidence suggests that prostaglandins, in low concentrations, sensitise tissues to several facets of the inflammatory response induced by other mediators (Ferreira & Vane 1974). Thus, inhibition of prostaglandin synthesis will appear to decrease the actions of other mediators such as bradykinin, histamine and 5-hydroxytryptamine.

The antipyretic analgesics which lack anti-inflammatory activity also inhibit prostaglandin synthetase, but they are relatively selective for the enzyme present in the brain. Paracetamol and aspirin are equipotent as inhibitors of brain prostaglandin synthetase, but paracetamol is ten times less active than aspirin against the spleen enzyme (Flower & Vane 1972). Thus, it may be that anti-inflammatory activity is brought about by inhibition of a prostaglandin synthetase, similar to that found in dog spleen, but dissimilar to that found in brain.

Antipyretic activity

Fevers, such as those produced by bacterial endotoxins or viruses, are probably caused by endogenous pyrogen derived from polymorphonuclear leucocytes. Endogenous pyrogens act directly upon the thermoregulatory neurones in the hypothalamus to increase the set-point temperature.

The principal site of the antipyretic activity of drugs, such as aspirin and paracetamol, would appear to be central since they antagonize the pyretic effects of intracerebrally injected leucocytic and bacterial pyrogens. However, aspirin has been shown to prevent release of endogenous pyrogen from the white cell, at least in the rabbit (Rawlins 1973). The central antipyretic action of aspirin-like drugs is neither a direct action upon the hypothalamus itself nor upon associated efferent pathways, as normal body temperature is t reduced and aspirin will not reduce the fever produced by local ɔoling of the hypothalamus (Cranston *et al.* 1970).

During fever of either pyrogenic or monoaminergic origin, considerable rises in prostaglandin E_1 concentration in the brain have been detected (Feldberg & Milton 1973). Indeed, prostaglandin E_1 is one of the most powerful pyretic agents yet examined and it appears to act on the same hypothalamic site as the pyrogens and pyretic monoamines. However, the antipyretic analgesics do not prevent the hyperthermia induced by intracerebral injections of prostaglandin E_1. Nevertheless, they do prevent the rise in prostaglandin concentration seen during fever and the time courses of antipyretic action and suppression of prostaglandin increases run parallel. Furthermore, Flower and Vane (1972) have demonstrated that both paracetamol and aspirin inhibit the enzyme prostaglandin synthetase in brain. By preventing prostaglandin synthesis the antipyretic analgesics could inhibit the generation of prostaglandin E type substances by pyrogens, a process necessary for an increase in the 'set-point' temperature.

Respiration and acid base balance

Only the salicylates amongst the antipyretic analgesic agents have any notable action upon respiration and acid base balance.

The actions of increasing doses of aspirin upon these parameters are summarized in Fig. 4.1.

Full therapeutic doses of aspirin uncouple oxidative phosphorylation in skeletal muscle resulting in increased oxygen consumption and carbon dioxide production. The increase in CO_2 production stimulates respiration so that the plasma PCO_2 is unchanged. However, in these circumstances, the patient has enhanced sensitivity to the production of respiratory acidosis by drugs which lower the respiratory response to carbon dioxide, for example, morphine, barbiturates.

As the plasma concentration of salicylate increases, it gains access to the medulla and stimulates respiration directly. This action of the salicylates predominates over the effects of carbon dioxide and thus the plasma PCO_2 falls. The respiratory alkalosis so formed is quickly compensated by renal excretion of bicarbonate accompanied by sodium and potassium; plasma bicarbonate falls and pH returns towards normal values.

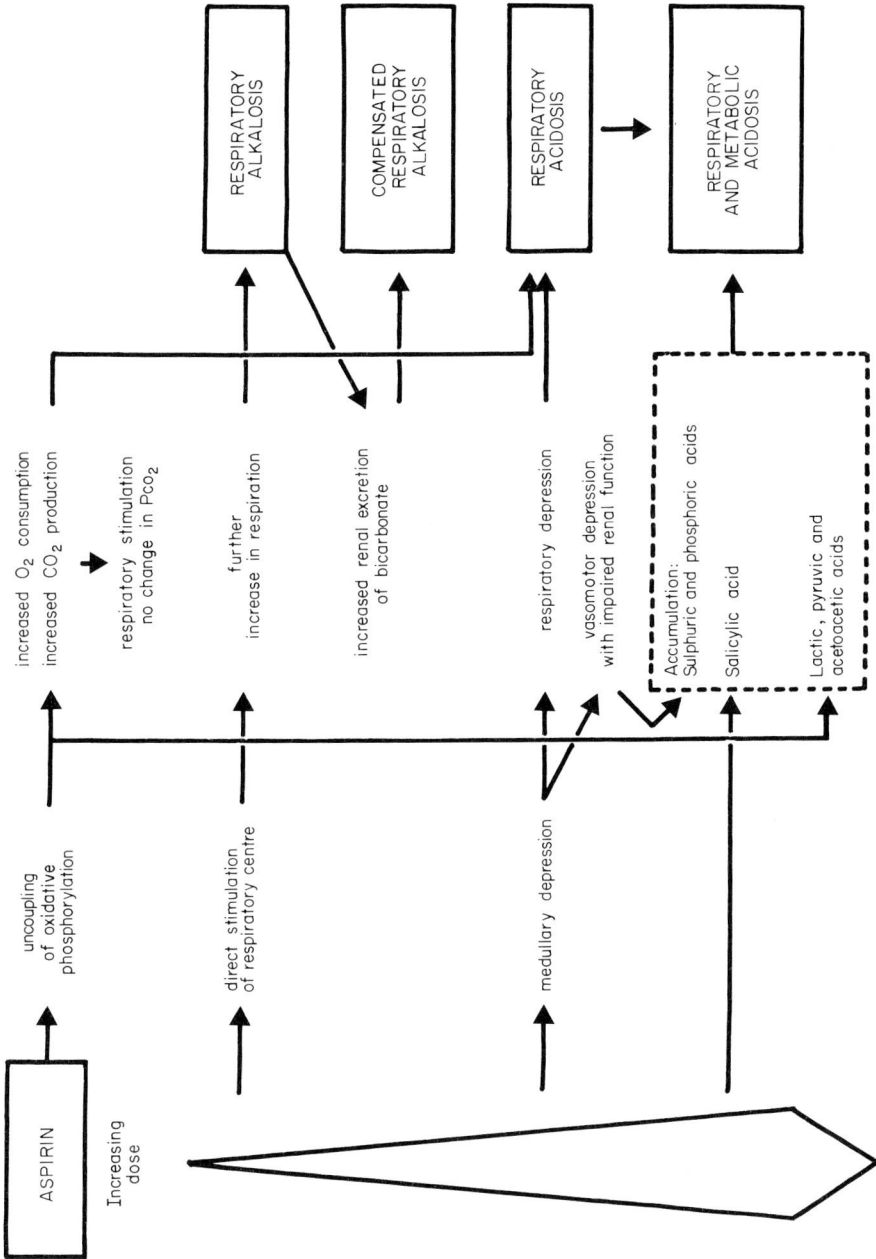

Fig. 4.1.

.er changes in acid base status occur when toxic doses are
.. High concentrations of salicylate depress respiration. This
.s the enhanced CO_2 production to outstrip alveolar excretion
at PCO_2 rises and pH falls. Since plasma bicarbonate is already
, the acid base state is an uncompensated respiratory acidosis.
Superimposed on this is a metabolic acidosis due to accumulation of
acids from three sources. In the presence of high doses of salicylates,
dissociation at plasma pH yields significant quantities of salicylic acid
and its derivatives. Concurrent with depression of the respiratory
centres is vasomotor depression. This may lead to impairment of
renal function and subsequent accumulation of strong acids of metabolic origin such as phosphoric and sulphuric acids. Finally, the
derangement of carbohydrate metabolism produced by the salicylates
results in an accumulation of organic acids such as pyruvic, lactic and
acetoacetic acids.

The treatment of these acid base problems and other signs of
salicylate poisoning have been reviewed by Hull (1973).

Hepatotoxicity

The salicylates appear to have very little action upon the liver even in
toxic doses. There is a fall in blood levels of prothrombin and fibrin-
ogen and some workers have suggested that this may indicate mild
liver dysfunction. The salicylates increase the volume of bile, but the
total cholate excretion is reduced.

However, not all antipyretic analgesics are as innocuous as the
salicylates with respect to the liver.

The first cases of hepatotoxicity from paracetamol overdosage
were reported in Britain in 1966 (Davidson & Eastham 1966, Thomson
& Prescott 1966). Proudfoot and Wright (1970) noted that cases of
paracetamol overdosage often exhibited liver damage although the
degree of hepatotoxicity did not appear to be directly related to the
dose of paracetamol ingested (Prescott & Wright 1973).

Animal work demonstrated that paracetamol was also
predictably hepatotoxic in the rat (Boyd & Berecsky 1966) and in
1973 a series of studies in rodents showed that the toxic effects of
paracetamol resided in an N-hydroxy metabolite. This metabolite
required cytochrome P450 for its formation and was capable of binding covalently to vital hepatic macromolecules (Mitchell *et al.*
1973 a, b, Jollow *et al.* 1973, Potter *et al.* 1973). The existence of a
hepatotoxic metabolite of paracetamol in man is supported by the

finding that previous consumption of enzyme inducing agents increases the hepatotoxicity of paracetamol (Wright & Prescott 1973). It seems that after therapeutic doses of paracetamol, this toxic metabolite is conjugated with liver glutathione and excreted as harmless cysteine and mercapturic acid conjugates of paracetamol. However, with toxic doses of paracetamol, the rate of production of the reactive toxic metabolite exceeds that of glutathione and the metabolite is left free to exert its cellular damage and death.

Animal experiments have confirmed that paracetamol produces a dose dependent depletion of glutathione and that the hepatotoxicity of paracetamol could be increased by glutathione depleting agents such as diethyl maleate. More importantly, paracetamol toxicity could be decreased by the administration of glutathione precursors or SH donors such as cysteine and cysteamine.

In view of these findings, trials to determine the effectiveness of cysteamine in treating paracetamol overdoses in man were instigated. Preliminary studies by Prescott *et al.* (1974) were promising. However cysteamine has some unpleasant side effects and in a later study L-methionine and D-penicillamine were examined as possible alternatives to cysteamine (Prescott *et al.* 1977). D-penicillamine was without protective effects in the dosage used and it appeared to enhance the nephrotoxicity of paracetamol. L-methionine, whilst effectively preventing liver damage in some cases of paracetamol overdose, inexplicably failed in others. Only cysteamine was effective in all cases treated provided that it was given within 10 hours of the paracetamol ingestion. Administration of cysteamine more than 12 hours after ingestion was ineffective and potentially dangerous (Prescott *et al.* 1977).

Despite the undoubted success of cysteamine in the treatment of paracetamol overdosage in the hands of Prescott and colleagues, Douglas *et al.* (1976) had less satisfactory results. Whilst some of the signs of liver damage were less in patients given cysteamine, one patient out of 18 died and the toxic effects of paracetamol upon kidney and pancreas were not improved.

Indeed, Dixon (1976) suggested that many of the fatalities obtained with paracetamol were not due primarily to hepatotoxicity. Whilst these findings are at variance with those of other workers their importance in the management of paracetamol overdosage requires that a re-evaluation of paracetamol toxicity should be made (Lesna *et al.* 1976).

Analgesic nephropathy

The possible association between prolonged consumption of analgesic mixtures and kidney damage has been studied extensively since
the early 1950s.

The patient suffering from chronic analgesic mixture toxicity is
characterized by a high incidence of gastro-intestinal disturbances
(including peptic ulceration), anaemia, methaemoglobinaemia,
splenomegaly and renal damage. The patient is more often female
than male and may have a history of urinary tract infections.

The kidney lesions are primarily papillary necrosis with secondary interstitial nephritis. Initially, the injury is manifest as a reduced
tubular function and concentrating ability. This may progress to
renal insufficiency unless the abuse of analgesic mixtures stops.

Originally, phenacetin was implicated as the nephrotoxic agent as
it was common to all analgesic mixtures. However, it has been argued
that other drugs present in analgesic mixtures may be nephrotoxic.
Indeed, Prescott (1965) demonstrated in volunteers that aspirin in
high doses for a relative short period (3·6 g daily) caused more kidney
damage than either phenacetin, caffeine or paracetamol. More prolonged administration studies in animals and man have failed to
produce conclusive results (Abel 1971). Animal work has not been
consistently reproducible and studies in man are complicated by the
reluctance of patients to admit their total consumption of analgesics.
However, it would appear that renal problems are more often
reported after aspirin phenacetin mixtures than with either drug
alone (Murray & Goldberg 1975).

It must be pointed out that only a minority of patients who con-
sume analgesic mixtures to excess develop nephropathy, although a
recent survey has shown that 12 per cent of cases of chronic renal
failure could be attributed to analgesic abuse (Cove-Smith & Knapp
1978).

There are striking differences in the regional distribution of the
incidence of analgesic nephropathy. This has led to the suggestion
that some people may have a genetic predisposition to analgesic
nephropathy or that local contaminants in the commercially available analgesics might be the cause. Analgesics may increase the
susceptibility to urinary tract infections or alternatively urinary tract
infections may increase the likelihood of damage to the kidney by
analgesic agents.

All that seems clear is that prolonged consumption of large quantities of analgesics is hazardous and should be discouraged unless adequately supervised.

Gastrointestinal effects

With the exception of phenacetin and paracetamol, most of the antipyretic analgesics have been shown to cause epigastric pain, nausea and vomiting, gastric bleeding and ulceration.

In a recent study, Levy (1974) found that there were significant correlations between patients admitted to hospital with gastric bleeding or peptic ulcer and regular aspirin consumption. Indeed, many clinical studies have shown that a high proportion of patients with upper gastrointestinal haemorrhage take aspirin regularly (Paulus & Whitehouse 1973).

The effects of the anti-inflammatory, antipyretic analgesics upon the gastric mucosa appear to be local. It is only demonstrable upon oral administration, there is a correlation between drug blood levels and gastric damage and the effects can be potentiation by prior ingestion of alcohol (Paulus & Whitehouse 1973). The pH of the stomach would also appear to be critical as less gastric irritation occurs in achlorhydric patients, and Leonards and Levy (1969) have demonstrated that aspirin induced blood loss is reduced by administration of the aspirin in a buffered solution.

The mechanism by which the gastric erosion occurs is debatable. It has been suggested that the secretion of a protective mucus is inhibited by these agents or that the drugs cause precipitations of a protective glyco-protein (Paulus & Whitehouse 1973).

All the antipyretic analgesics that cause gastric irritation have marked anti-inflammatory properties which have been attributed to inhibition of peripheral prostaglandin synthetase. Thus, it is not surprising that a possible link between inhibition of prostaglandin synthesis and gastric irritation has been proposed (Ferreira & Vane 1974). It was suggested that prostaglandins in some way protected the gastric mucosa from damage, thus inhibition of prostaglandin synthesis would make the mucosa susceptible to damage.

Several possible protective mechanisms for the prostaglandins have been postulated. Protaglandin E_1 inhibits gastric secretion, so locally released prostaglandin could be a 'braking' mechanism to prevent hyperacidity. Prostaglandins also increase blood flow to the gastric mucosa and thus removal of this effect could lead to inadequate mucosal perfusion and perhaps necrosis (Bennett *et al.* 1973). A final possibility is that inhibition of prostaglandin synthesis could lead to a build up of precursors such as arachidonic acid which then cause gastric irritation.

Hypersensitivity reactions

Aspirin is the antipyretic analgesic most often involved in hypersensitive reactions and cross sensitivity with other salicylates or the para-amino phenol derivatives is uncommon. However, many aspirin hypersensitive patients are also hypersensitive to another anti-inflammatory agent, indomethacin.

Studies in the United States (Chafee & Settipane 1974, Settipane, Chafee & Klein 1974) have suggested that the incidence of aspirin intolerance is as high as 0·9 per cent in normal subjects and 4·3 per cent in asthmatics.

Sensitivity to aspirin may be manifest as rhinitis, skin rashes, asthma, angioneurotic oedema and laryngeal spasm. Concurrent gastrointestinal disturbances are also common. Samter and Beers (1968) observed that aspirin hypersensitivity was not similar to other allergic phenomena and suggested that a non-immunological mechanism might be involved. Samter and Beer (1968) suggested that this could be an increased sensitivity of areas like the nasal mucosa to pharmacologically active peptides such as bradykinin. This theory is interesting in that the opposite mechanism, i.e. decreased sensitivity to peptides etc., due to inhibition of prostaglandin synthesis, has been proposed for the anti-inflammatory actions of aspirin (see p. 72).

Whilst many of the aspirin hypersensitivity responses are amenable to treatment with sympathomimetics such as adrenaline, the bronchial asthma is sometimes refractory to therapy.

Chapter 5 · Antipyretic Analgesics
II. Individual agents and mixtures

Aspirin is the standard antipyretic analgesic, against which all others are compared. Absorption of non-ionized aspirin occurs in the stomach, but this is reduced if the pH is raised. Aspirin is also absorbed from the intestine.

In both the intestine and the circulation, aspirin is rapidly hydrolysed to salicylic acid. Salicylate is extensively protein bound (50–80 percent) but aspirin itself is only protein-bound to a limited extent. Distribution to body tissues is rapid with the highest concentrations of salicylate occurring in the kidney, liver, heart and lungs.

The biological half life of aspirin was found to be 2 to 3 hours after a single dose, but up to 10 hours after multiple doses (Cummings & Martin 1968).

The metabolites of aspirin, mainly salicylic acid, salicyluric acid, gentisic acid and glucuronides are excreted in the urine (Fig. 5.1). The proportion of free salicylic acid is very variable and depends to a great extent upon urinary pH, particularly in the alkaline range. Mean salicylate clearance is increased 4 times when the urinary pH increases from 6 to 8.

A number of special aspirin formulations have been produced in an effort to improve on the absorption and elimination of aspirin resulting in a more intense, earlier and more prolonged analgesic effect, as well as to reduce the dyspepsia and blood loss sometimes associated with aspirin administration. Whilst some of these preparations, notably soluble and buffered aspirin, produce higher salicylate blood levels, there have been no clinical trials which have demonstrated any concurrent increase in analgesic activity (Beaver 1965). However, small particle size and the incorporation of an antacid have produced significantly less gastric bleeding (Györy & Stiel 1968, Leonards & Levy 1969).

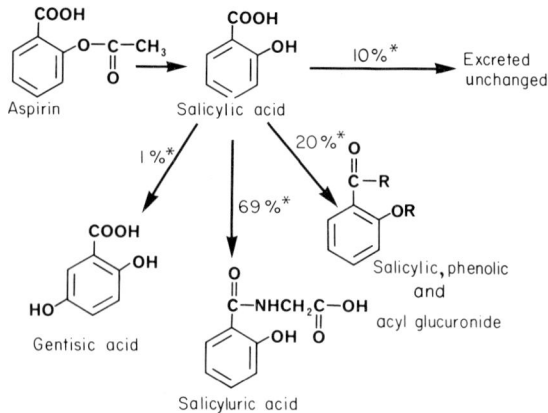

*Applies to excretion in acid urine

Fig. 5.1. Structure and metabolism of aspirin and salicylic acid.

Acetylsalicylic acid's efficacy in the treatment of mild to moderate pain of various aetiologies has been demonstrated convincingly on numerous occasions (Beaver 1965). In a comparison of 9 analgesic drugs marketed in the United States, none was found to be superior to aspirin for the treatment of cancer pain assessed to be mild to moderate in character (Moertal *et al.* 1972).

Aspirin is valuable for the relief of certain types of pain such as headache, arthritis, dysmenorrhoea, neuralgia and myalgia. Its anti-inflammatory actions are useful in the treatment of rheumatoid arthritis and despite the advent of newer drugs, salicylates are still considered the drug of choice for this condition.

Aspirin is also an effective antipyretic for cases in which fever is deleterious. This effect of aspirin is nonspecific and does not influence the course of the underlying disease (Done 1959).

Once absorbed, acetylsalicylic acid is rapidly hydrolysed to salicylic acid in the plasma, liver the erythrocytes and more slowly in the synovial fluid. It was originally thought that the pharmacological activity of aspirin resided in the salicylic acid metabolite, but it is now clear that the ester has activity in its own right (Collier 1969).

In view of the millions of aspirin tablets ingested each year, it is a remarkably non-toxic drug; however, certain side effects are worthy of note. Most common is gastrointestinal bleeding and irritation, which has been discussed elsewhere (p. 79). In large doses, salicylates reduce prothrombin levels and this is preventable by the administration of vitamin K. The prolongation of prothrombin time is mainly due to a decrease in Factor VII (proconvertin), the stable prothrombin conversion factor (Quick & Clesceri 1960). The effects of salicylates on prothrombin time are enhanced by fever and summate with the effects of the bishydroxycoumarin derivatives. Indeed, it has been suggested that the salicylates and the coumarins reduce prothrombin time by the same mechanism, i.e. interference of the role of vitamin K in prothrombin synthesis.

However, the gastrointestinal bleeding does not seem to be related to this action of the drug in most cases, as the prothrombinopenic effect is seen only with high doses of aspirin. More important is the effects of aspirin on platelet adhesiveness. Doses as low as 650 mg double bleeding time in man for several days and this is associated with a block of the adhesion of platelets to connective tissue and collagen fibres (Mustard & Packman 1970). This property of aspirin has led to several potential therapeutic uses of the drug. The prophylactic administration of aspirin has been found useful in preventing venous thrombosis and pulmonary embolism. It is also undergoing studies in the prophylaxis of coronary thrombosis (Woodbury & Fingle 1975).

PARACETAMOL

Paracetamol, the major metabolite of phenacetin, is an antipyretic analgesic with negligible anti-inflammatory activity. Although generally well absorbed from the gastrointestinal tract, paracetamol absorption as low as 25 per cent has been demonstrated in healthy persons (Gwilt *et al.* 1963). Paracetamol is 25 per cent protein bound and about 3 per cent of the drug is excreted unchanged in the urine. The remainder (80 per cent) is conjugated in the liver with predominantly glucuronic acid and to a small extent with sulphuric acid. These conjugates are excreted in the urine (Fig. 5.2).

As an analgesic, paracetamol is approximately equipotent with aspirin (Parkhouse & Hallinon 1967, Moertal *et al.* 1972). However, due to its lack of anti-inflammatory activity, it is a less useful drug for alleviation of the pain associated with inflammatory conditions such as active rheumatoid arthritis (Hajnal *et al.* 1959). The antipyretic activity of paracetamol is also similar to that of aspirin (Colgan & Mintz 1957).

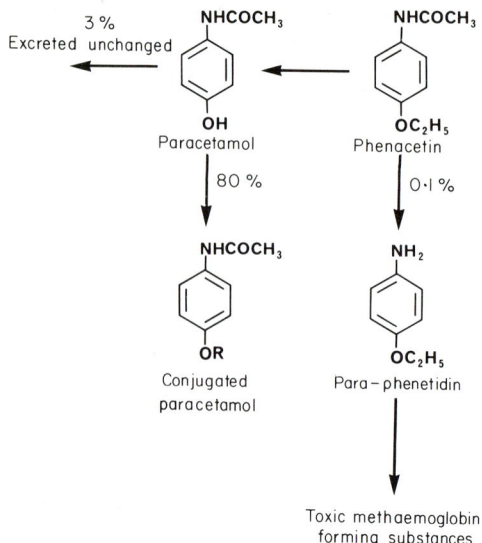

Fig. 5.2. Structure and metabolism of phenacetin and paracetamol.

Paracetamol does not cause gastric irritation or the blood loss characteristic of aspirin and it has not been associated with any coagulation defects (Beaver 1965). Unlike its parent compound, phenacetin, paracetamol is rarely associated with methaemoglobinaemia and has not been implicated in haemolytic anaemia. Indeed, unless the drug is abused, side effects are rarely seen. Since patients exhibiting allergy to aspirin are rarely cross sensitive to paracetamol, in recent years paracetamol has been considered the most reasonable alternative to aspirin for the treatment of pain not associated with an active inflammatory condition.

However, despite paracetamol's apparent freedom from side effects in therapeutic doses, overdosage may produce potentially fatal liver damage (see p. 76). Fatalities have occurred with doses as low as 15 g (30 tablets) and since the signs of liver damage become obvious only some days after the overdose, the serious nature of the poisoning may not be appreciated until the condition is untreatable.

PHENACETIN

In man, phenacetin is readily absorbed from the gastrointestinal tract and is rapidly biotransformed to paracetamol, which is subsequently conjugated and excreted in the urine (Brodie & Axelrod 1948 a & b,

1949). It was suggested by these workers that paracetamol may be the active metabolite by which phenacetin and the related compound acetanilid exert their analgesic and antipyretic actions. However, in 1966, Conney *et al.* demonstrated that enhancement of the rate of metabolism of phenacetin to paracetamol was associated with a decrease in the antipyretic activity of phenacetin in rats. This suggests that the parent compound may possess activity in its own right, independent of metabolism to paracetamol.

A trace of phenacetin is deacetylated in man to form p-phenetidin which is the precursor of acetophenetidin (Fig. 5.2) which in turn is responsible for methaemoglobin formation (Brodie & Axelrod 1949). However, there is no evidence that the small quantities of methaemoglobin formed by even repeated therapeutic doses of phenacetin have any deleterious effects. Nevertheless, some degree of tissue anoxia can be expected after large overdoses of phenacetin (Beaver 1965).

Whilst phenacetin has no marked anti-inflammatory or antirheumatic activity it has similar analgesic activity to aspirin in post partum pain (Lasagna, Davis & Pearson 1967). In contrast to aspirin, it causes no gastric blood loss or irritation to mucosal surfaces (Beaver 1965). In recent years, it has been available only in combination with aspirin or other antipyretic analgesic agents. However, the recent controversy about nephrotoxicity (see p. 78) has lead to its deletion from most of these preparations.

MEFENAMIC ACID AND FLUFENAMIC ACID

Mefenamic acid and flufenamic acid are anthranilic acid derivatives which have a spectrum of activity similar to aspirin. Suggested indications include relief of mild to moderate pain and, more specifically in the case of flufenamic acid, pain associated with rheumatic conditions. Mefenamic acid is also recommended for pyrexia in children.

Although an effective analgesic, the gastrointestinal side effects of mefenamic acid may prove troublesome (Moertal *et al.* 1972). Diarrhoea may occur with ordinary doses and necessitates the immediate cessation of medication. Dyspepsia, gastrointestinal bleeding and ulceration have all been reported and the drug is contra-indicated in patients showing evidence of intestinal ulceration.

Agranulocytosis, thrombocytopenic purpura, megaloblastic anaemia and pancytopenia have also been reported and the manufacturers recommend that blood studies should be carried out during long term mefenamic acid therapy. Furthermore, mefenamic acid should be used with caution in subjects with renal impairment as animal studies with prolonged high doses of the drug have suggested enhanced toxicity in these circumstances.

Both mefenamic acid and flufenamic acid have been shown to prolong prothrombin time in patients treated with coumarin anti-coagulants. However, there is little evidence that mefenamic acid or indeed flufenamic acid affects the blood clotting mechanism when given alone.

There is no evidence that either mefenamic or flufenamic acid is superior to any of the established analgesics (e.g. Barnardo *et al.* 1966). Thus, in view of possible toxic side effects and the high cost of the compounds, the rationale for their continued use has been seriously questioned (Moertal *et al.* 1972, Goodman & Gilman 1975).

SALICYLAMIDE

Salicylamide is not a salicylate as it lacks a free carboxyl group, neither is it converted to salicylate on administration (Mandel *et al.* 1952). Whilst salicylamide appears to be a more potent anti-nociceptive agent than aspirin in animals (Way *et al.* 1953), clinical studies have provided grounds for scepticism concerning salicylamide's analgesic activity in man although it has been suggested that the drug may have a small early analgesic effect which is rapidly dissipated (Beaver 1965). Salicylamide is also inferior to aspirin as an antipyretic agent (Borovsky 1960).

In contrast to aspirin, salicylamide neither increases prothrombin time (Quick & Clesceri 1960) nor causes gastric bleeding (Wood 1963). In overdosage, salicylamide produces central nervous system depression and the hyperpnoea and acid base disturbances associated with salicylism are not observed (Done 1959).

However, in view of its doubtful efficacy, salicylamide has been withdrawn from most pharmacopoeias, but may be found in some 'over the counter' preparations.

SODIUM SALICYLATE

Sodium salicylate had already been extensively used before the introduction of aspirin in 1899. Although it was originally thought that the actions of aspirin were due to conversion to salicylate in the blood, a number of trials have shown convincingly that the analgesic action of sodium salicylate is inferior to equimolar doses of aspirin (Frey 1961, Stockman 1913). Furthermore, Seed (1965) demonstrated that sodium salicylate was inferior to aspirin as an antipyretic agent. These findings are particularly interesting since sodium salicylate is absorbed faster and gives higher salicylate blood levels than do equivalent doses of aspirin (Hogben *et al.* 1957, Wiegand & Perry 1962). It also illustrates the dubious validity of trying to associate salicylate blood levels with analgesic activity.

Chapter 6 · Controlled Clinical Trials
of Analgesic Drugs

'If we take a patient afflicted with a malady, and we alter his conditions of life, either by dieting him, or by putting him to bed, or by
administering to him a drug, or by performing on him an operation,
we are performing an experiment. And if we are scientifically minded
we should record the results. Before concluding that the change for
better or for worse in the patient is due to the specific treatment
employed, we must ascertain whether the results can be repeated a
significant number of times in similar patients, whether the result was
merely due to the natural history of the disease or in other words to
the lapse of time, or whether it was due to some other factor which
was necessarily associated with the therapeutic measure in question.'
(Pickering 1949).

General principles

1. Control

The principle of control implies that a drug or method of treatment
will be fairly compared with an alternative. It is not sufficient to say
that a certain drug, given in certain circumstances, is effective. Apart
from the problem of defining what is meant by effective there is the
possibility that other factors, including nature itself, may contribute
more to relief than the medication. To compare the drug against an
alternative given in exactly the same circumstances thus helps to define
the sources of variation in outcome.

(a) i. COMPARISON WITH A STANDARD DRUG

It is of no interest to discover that a new analgesic is better than a
placebo. It must bear comparison with the best known alternative. In

the case of a narcotic analgesic and an antipyretic analgesic the standards of comparison will normally be morphine and aspirin respectively.

It is essential in such comparisons to use comparable doses, and a pilot trial may be necessary to determine these. Many trials have failed or misled because it subsequently became clear that the chosen dose of the drug in question was too low.

Once the relative potency of the new drug to the standard is approximately known, the most comprehensive and informative type of trial to conduct, if feasible, is a logarithmic dose-response study, including a standard of comparison. Within the clinically effective dose range it is to be expected that the increasing responses to drug doses which rise in logarithmic ratio will lie on a straight line. At least three points should therefore be available. For example, if a new analgesic has approximately the same potency as pethidine, a clinical trial might be designed using 25 mg, 50 mg and 100 mg (i.e. 25×2^0, 25×2^1 and 25×2^2 mg) compared to 10 mg morphine and, if indicated, a placebo. Such a trial may give useful information about whether it is worthwhile using the largest dose, whether the smallest dose is significantly better than a placebo and what dose is comparable to 10 mg of morphine. It may give additional information about whether the duration of action is significantly prolonged by increasing the dose and whether there appears to be a threshold for the development of side effects. An illustration of such a trial using pethidine as a standard, is shown in Fig. 6.1. (Parkhouse & Wright 1968).

ii. COMPARISON WITH A PLACEBO

There are two main reasons for wishing to compare an analgesic with a placebo. The first is to establish the background level of improvement which may be expected without any specific pharmacological effect. This is likely to vary considerably in different situations, for example in simple headache as compared to the intractable pain of malignant disease. Egbert *et al.* (1964) and Roe (1963) have noted the profound effects of explanation and reassurance in reducing the need for post-operative narcotics. Saunders (1966) and others who work in terminal care units have stressed the value of social, religious and psychological support in controlling pain.

Improvement occurring without the use of a pharmacologically active agent may result either from the psychological effect of giving a

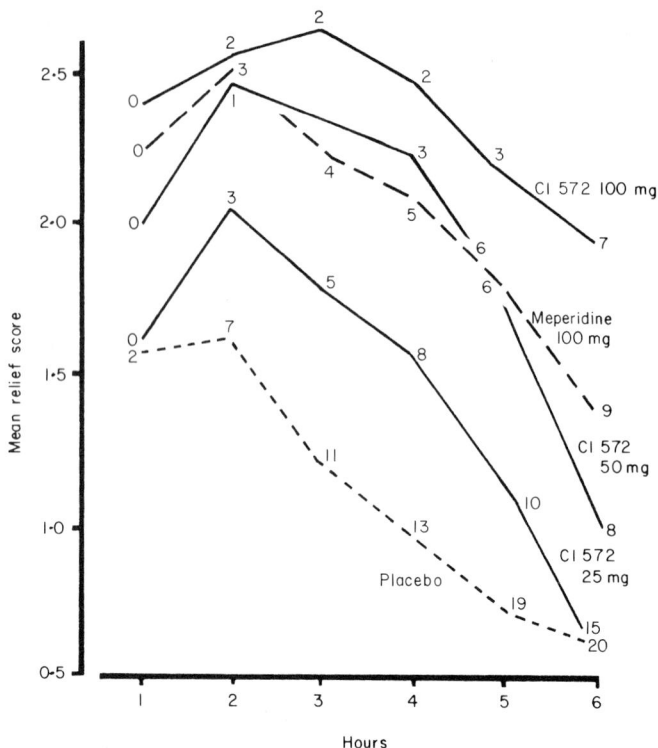

Fig. 6.1. Scores for pain relief in groups of patients at hourly intervals after administration of three doses of the analgesic Cl 572 (Parke, Davis), 100 mg pethidine (meperidine) and a placebo. The increasing effectiveness of logarithmically rising doses of the analgesic is seen clearly, as is the comparability of 50 mg to 100 mg pethidine. The numbers against each point on each curve show how many of the patients in each group had already received a further analgesic at the time indicated. This gives additional information about efficacy and duration of action, particularly in regard to the placebo. (Originally published *C. M. A. Journal*, **99**: 887–891.)

placebo or from other causes. To separate these it would be necessary, strictly speaking, to include placebo-treated and completely untreated groups of patients in a trial. This may be of value in situations where it is unclear whether pain resolves spontaneously or responds principally to the induced expectation of relief. For most practical purposes, however, it is unnecessary to make such distinctions in analgesic studies, and it is preferable not to compound the ethical difficulties of withholding some form of treatment.

Attempts have been made to define the level of response to be expected from giving a placebo and some constancy for this has been claimed (Jellinek 1946, Beecher 1955). Related efforts have been made to analyse the reported severity of pain and the demand for analgesics in relation to personality and other characteristics of the individual patient (Lasagna *et al.* 1954, Boyle & Parbrook 1977). There is a striking contrast between the consistent averages of sufficiently large groups of patients and the very different behaviour of individuals within each group, and this must colour any interpretation of the reported incidence of 'placebo reactors'.

The definition of a 'placebo reactor' rests upon the criterion of relief (Parkhouse 1963); it is no more reasonable, and no less, to describe a man as a placebo reactor than to describe him as being 'relieved', without qualification, by morphine. It remains to be added that relief following the administration of an active drug is not necessarily the result of a direct pharmacological action; for 'within every active drug there lies a placebo'.

The second reason for using a placebo is to discover whether a clinical trial is sensitive enough to be capable of detecting significant differences. When a comparison between two active drugs shows no statistically significant difference, this may mean that the drugs are closely similar in effect, or that the method of testing was not sufficiently sensitive to reveal a difference. This is a particular problem with subjective phenomena like pain, where the precision of the available methods of measurement is not easily tested. The ability to distinguish clearly a placebo from active drugs adds greatly to the credibility of a trial. It is by no means clear, however, that sufficient reproducibility can be claimed to justify the contention that, once this has been done, a placebo may be omitted from subsequent trials conducted in the same way. There thus remains an ethical problem.

(b) THE PATIENT 'AS HIS OWN CONTROL'

If each patient in a trial receives only one of the treatments concerned, which may include a placebo, there will naturally be difficulty in comparing the resulting assessments. If the first patient's opinion of drug *A* is more favourable than the second patient's opinion of drug *B* this may signify either a difference in the drugs or in the patients' responses to pain and to treatment in general. If each patient receives both drugs in turn, both can give a comparative assessment of the two treatments. Furthermore, if the first patient receives drug *A* followed by drug *B* and the second patient receives drug *B* followed by drug *A*, due allowance can be made in evaluating their opinions for any natural tendency for pain to increase or diminish with time or for any persistence of the effect of either of the drugs.

This use of the patient 'as his own control' is the basis of the 'crossover' type of design, and the derivation of the term will be self-evident. It is an elementary refinement of technique which often confers obvious advantages. Many more complex refinements are possible, for example with four or five treatments each repeated on a number of occasions, but in most cases simple designs and simple methods are best, since they are least likely to be upset by the inevitable variations associated with clinical practice.

2. Elimination of bias

In any assessment, but particularly when subjective judgments are to be made, the greatest care is needed to avoid deliberate or unconscious prejudice for or against the outcome of a particular drug administration. The factors that may lead a patient or an observer to anticipate a favourable response, or the reverse, include foreknowledge of the drug to be given, preconceived views of its efficacy, nuances in the way it is presented and in the manner of enquiry about its effect, casual comment from ward staff, doctors or other patients and accumulation of experience from contemporary researchers or from previous cases in 'open' trial. Actual differences in response, apparently but not really due to the drug, may result from variations in general management of patients admitted on different days or to different units, and many other causes. Most of these points are obvious in principle, although in practice the difficulties may be more subtle; for example, in a study of post-operative vomiting it will be necessary to ensure that the same post-operative regime regarding food and drink is followed by patients in each treatment group (Riding 1960).

It should be stressed that the substitution of a supposedly objective measurement, such as vital capacity, for subjective assessment of pain relief does not remove the need for scrupulous care in the elimination of bias.

(a) RANDOMIZATION

There is no adequate substitute for complete randomization of the order in which different drugs or treatment regimes in any trial are assigned to successive patients. As indicated above, it is obviously not sufficient to take first a series of patients given one drug and then a series given the next alternative; nor is it enough to assign every second or third patient, or those admitted on every second or third day to each of two or three treatment groups. Once the number of treatment groups and the number of patients to be included in each group are decided, the allocation should, wherever possible, be completely random. Tables of random numbers or an equivalent device may be used for this purpose. This assignment must, of course, be in the hands of a person not directly concerned with administration or assessment. The only knowledge available to those actually conducting the trial should be that a code exists, indicating which drug will be given to each patient; in case of emergency, for example an unexpected adverse reaction, this code may be 'broken' but it should normally remain sealed until the trial is completed. The actual medications will be packaged individually, bearing the number of the patient to whom they are to be given, and will be identical in appearance and other relevant characteristics.

(b) THE MEANING OF 'DOUBLE BLIND'

The patient should be told about the study in which he is invited to participate, without being told what drugs are being compared. For example, he may be told that a study is being made of a number of different pain-relieving drugs, some of which may prove to be better than others. He is asked if he is willing to be given one, or some, of the drugs for the purpose of a study. No further information need usually be given about the specific nature of the medications, but if he asks about possible side effects or whether a placebo is included he should be answered honestly and as informatively as seems reasonable.

If the experimental design involves giving more than one dose, it is as well to say that the medications received may be identical or different. A neutral approach of this kind is the most likely to eliminate imaginative reporting and well-intentioned efforts to guess which drug is supposed to be the best.

Any person who is involved with the administering of the drugs, the general care of the patient or the assessment of effects must also be ignorant of what has been given. This mutual innocence, of both the giver and the receiver of each test drug, gives rise to the description of such trials as 'double blind'. But it is clear that many more than two people usually need to be 'blind' in order to preserve a strict immunity from bias; chance remarks are easily made in earshot of the patient or the observer. It is a good test if at the end of the trial those concerned are still unaware of the identity and dosage of the drugs used and are still unable to say how many treatment groups there were. Surprisingly often, in a good study, the person who has made the assessments is unsure at the end whether or not a placebo was used.

3. Definition of the problem

(a) WHAT QUESTION IS TO BE ANSWERED?

Only a small trial may be needed if a very specific question is to be resolved; for example, does pethidine cause dizziness in young adult male patients who are allowed out of bed post-operatively? No conclusions could be drawn, however, about the effect of the drug in children or in obstetric practice and it may well turn out that an attempt to relate the dizziness to hypotension, nausea, concurrent drug therapy and other factors would require a much larger study.

A critical question at the planning stage, therefore, is which patients are to be included or excluded, and how those included are to be grouped or classified.

With a sufficient number of patients included in a trial, it may be expected that many of the potentially relevant factors will, by chance, be fairly evenly distributed between the treatment groups. This should be demonstrated at the end and allowance must be made for discrepancies when evaluating the results. Alternatively, if certain factors are of particular importance, the trial should be planned in advance so that these are balanced out between the treatments. For example, in a comparison of analgesics in post-operative pain it would be important to know that the groups of patients given each of the drugs included roughly the same proportions of long operations, old people, men and women, and so forth, and it would need to be decided whether premedication and anaesthesia should be standardized, or allowed for, and what types of operation should be included.

When exclusions are kept to a minimum and quite large numbers of patients are included in a trial, it often happens that interesting information is obtained on more than one specific point. Conversely, the sequential trial is especially suited to a highly specific objective and if there is interest in two or three effects of the drugs concerned the sequential approach virtually requires two or three separate trials.

It is impossible to over-emphasize the importance of considering in advance what data are to be collected and what questions most need to be answered.

(b) WITH WHAT DEGREE OF PRECISION?

Decisions about excluding certain types of patients from a trial, or about attempting to balance out extraneous factors by random distribution among treatment groups, will affect the sensitiveness of a trial. The type of experimental design, for example the ability to give more than one drug to each patient, will also have an influence. In pain studies the fineness and number of gradations that are used in assessment have little effect on sensitivity; in all probability very little, if anything, is lost by using a simple distinction between relief and lack of relief as compared, for example, with a ten or twenty point scale which implies a degree of scientific precision in measurement that does not exist in reality.

If it is essential not to miss a significant difference, almost however small, between two drugs, a large number of patients may have to be studied. In analgesic trials this is very rarely the case. It is important to distinguish between a *statistically* significant difference, which may be satisfying to the investigator and the drug manufacturer, and a *clinically* significant difference, which is what matters to the patient. Generally speaking, quite simple trials are capable of revealing any differences between analgesic drugs that are likely to be of clinical importance.

(c) WITH WHAT RISK OF ERROR?

In any controlled trial there are two risks to be considered: the risk of mistakenly believing that a significant difference has been found when in fact none exists, and the risk of failing to detect a significant difference which is actually present. These are commonly described as Type 1 and Type 2 error, respectively, and their probabilities are written as α and β. Circumstances will indicate which, if either, is more important.

Bearing in mind what would be an acceptable risk of each of these errors, it is possible to estimate on statistical grounds the numbers of patients that need to be studied. Simple charts have been designed for this purpose in conventional trials (Clark & Downie 1966).

For sequential trials the framework is set up from the outset on the basis of what risks of error are acceptable. The number of cases is not pre-determined in a sequential trial, and the study may be discontinued as soon as the boundary of the chart is crossed by continuous plotting of results as they are obtained, thus indicating that the desired level of 'statistical significance' has been attained. There are obvious ethical advantages in such a design, and it avoids the occasional embarrassment of finding, at the end of an extensive conventional study, that the significance level of the differences shown is far in excess of what was actually needed for clinical purposes.

The investigator must have a clear understanding of the degree of sensitivity that he requires in his study, and it must be remembered that a trial which is primarily meant to answer one question will probably be much less sensitive in relation to other questions. This is especially important in regard to side effects. Drugs which nowadays reach the stage of clinical trial are likely to show a very low incidence of side effects and it is not therefore reasonable to expect a limited trial to reveal these. Indeed, the design of most trials tends to exclude any patients considered particularly likely to show adverse reactions.

Practical considerations

1. The pilot trial

It is sometimes highly desirable to begin by carrying out a small 'open' trial (i.e. not double blind) in order to establish the relative potency of the drugs to be compared. Such a pilot trial may also reveal unexpected side effects, especially if high doses are contemplated, and may help to test methods of assessment. Other necessary information can be obtained, such as the acceptability of the proposed investigation to patients and staff, the time span over which assessments need to be made (i.e. the duration of drug action) and the numbers of suitable patients available. Time spent on a small preliminary study may thus avoid many errors and heartaches at a later stage. One problem, however, is that it may then be difficult to carry out a genuinely 'double blind' full-scale trial in the same institution.

2. Ethical problems

(a) USE OF PLACEBOS

In some clinical situations, the use of a placebo is utterly impossible in practice. The most obvious example would be the assessment of a new inhalation anaesthetic agent as the sole means of pain relief during surgery. There is, however, always an ethical problem in using a placebo for patients who are in pain. There are different shades of opinion, and clearly the situation is not the same in severe cancer pain as in mild musculo-skeletal discomfort.

In the United Kingdom there would be general agreement that a placebo should be used, not as a matter of routine, but for specific and justifiable reasons, as already indicated. Furthermore, the trial should be arranged so that any patient who is not adequately relieved of pain after the given drug has had time to take effect may be given an analgesic of known efficacy without delay. Apart from its ethical unacceptability, insistence that all patients, including those who receive a placebo, must wait at least four hours before receiving a further analgesic would result in loss of valuable clinical information from those patients who patently failed to obtain relief. It is, in a sense, tantamount to 'screening in' placebo reactors. Likewise, attempts to identify placebo reactors so that they may be 'screened out' of a trial in the hope of improving discrimination will also result in loss of valuable information.

(b) ELIMINATION OF BIAS

This is made difficult when unusual or technically complex methods of pain relief are to be compared with more conventional methods. For example, inhalation or epidural analgesia for post-operative pain requires increased attention to the patient and cannot be used 'blind'. A truly unbiased study of epidural block compared with morphine would require that each patient had an epidural catheter in place and also received intramuscular injections, a placebo being given in some cases through the catheter and in others intramuscularly. This illustrates how the desire for absolute control must sometimes be tempered by awareness of what is ethically justifiable and clinically practicable.

3. Clinical circumstances

A method which depends on complex measurement may exhaust or confuse some patients, whilst drawing useful information from others. A trial which requires every subject to receive, in random order, each of five or six drugs or mixtures may have convincing theoretical advantages in a study of chronic pain, but if it happens that a considerable number of patients, for various reasons, have failed to complete the sequence a statistical analysis may be virtually impossible. Nothing is to be gained by giving drugs to patients when they are not really in pain in order to increase the number of cases studied, or to comply with the requirements of a protocol. Complex multi-dose studies are, however, sometimes valuable, and there are situations in which a regular schedule of analgesic dosage has advantages, despite fluctuations in pain intensity. The type of assessment that can be made in hospital over a short time scale may be quite impossible for ambulatory patients in a long-term trial. The numbers of cases available for study will be much greater with some forms of pain than others.

In short, the investigator must always be prepared to adapt his plans to the clinical circumstances.

Methods of assessment

Pain is a personal experience which may show itself externally in various ways. It is thus possible to seek evidence about pain either by asking the patient to record or describe his feelings, or by looking for indications of discomfort. If the performance of some movement or test provokes or exacerbates pain, this can perhaps be used as an objective index of the severity of the pain. It may not always be ethically acceptable deliberately to cause pain for this purpose, but in many circumstances there is positive benefit to the patient. Ability to move the limbs in arthritis, or to cough after upper abdominal surgery is important, and the objective testing of this ability not only gives an indication of pain relief but encourages the patient to exploit that relief to his own advantage.

1. Self-assessment

(a) 'ABSOLUTE'

Only the patient knows precisely what his pain is like, and the concomitant suffering belongs primarily to him. In assessing severity and relief of pain it is simplest, therefore, to ask the patient for his own judgment.

Qualitative description may be helpful although often, in Virginia Woolf's frequently quoted words, 'language at once runs dry'. Keele (1948) suggested the use of a 'pain chart' on which the patient could record the severity of his pain, against an arbitrary scale, at intervals of time. More recently, a white card bearing a 10 cm line has been used for the same purpose. The patient is asked to imagine that the right hand end of the line represents the most severe pain imaginable and that the left hand end represents pain so slight as to be only just perceptible; he is then asked to mark on this line whereabouts his existing pain lies. Cards can be presented to the patient at various time intervals; they can be left at the bedside or provided for home use. Most patients find the method easy to understand, after a little explanation, and useful data can be obtained. An imaginary pain scale from 0 to 100 has also been suggested. If the cards are presented dispassionately or, preferably, if the patient is left to mark them entirely on his own, the resulting information is the nearest possible approach to the personal and unmodified feeling of the sufferer. Revill *et al.* (1976) have recently assessed the variability of this technique and a fuller discussion, with a note of caution, is given by Nicholson (1978) and Maxwell (1978).

(b) COMPARATIVE

The general principle of using the patient 'as his own control' has already been discussed. It may be applied to assessment simply by asking the patients to say which of two or more analgesics, or regimes they prefer; the method has been used in chronic musculo-skeletal pain and in comparing inhalation agents for obstetrical analgesia. A classical example was the study which Seward (1949) carried out, with the help of the statistician D. J. Finney, to compare 50 per cent nitrous oxide in air, 75 per cent nitrous oxide with oxygen and 0·5 per cent trichloroethylene in air. Each patient received two of the three mixtures and was asked to say which she thought more effective;

there were 50 patients in each group and the numbers expressing such opinions were as shown in the following table:

| Mixtures compared | | Better | | Equal |
(a)	(b)	(a)	(b)	
50% Nitrous-oxide/air	75% Nitrous-oxide/oxygen	0	49	1
50% Nitrous-oxide/air	Trichloroethylene/air	0	45	5
75% Nitrous-oxide/oxygen	Trichloroethylene/air	14	12	24

It is immediately obvious that trichloroethylene and 75 per cent nitrous oxide were indistinguishable to the patients, but that both were preferred to 50 per cent nitrous oxide. This is an excellent example of the way in which good design and sound method can be so combined that statistical analysis is unnecessary.

Many other uses of comparison by the patient are possible. In long-continued treatment of chronic pain, for example in arthritis, Batterman (1965) suggested the expedient of changing from one treatment to the other without the patient's knowledge and merely observing how soon the difference was noticed. With proper planning, a good deal can be learned in this way about placebo responses, persistence of drug effects, clinically worthwhile differences between one analgesic regime and another, and about variations between patients in their tolerance and preference for different drugs.

2. Use of trained observers

H. K. Beecher was probably the first person to suggest the employment of a 'neutral observer' in the assessment of pain (Keats *et al.* 1950). He originally meant neither a doctor nor a nurse, but in practice most studies have used trained nurses as observers.

The question of how much an observer can legitimately pass judgment on the severity of another person's pain, and the quality of its relief, has been widely debated and continues to arouse strong feelings. It must first of all be recognized that even in a completely 'double blind' trial, the dialogue between patient and observer is one between human beings. Rarely will any patient give a clear and unprompted description of his pain as moderate, or severe; never will any observer, however 'neutral', fail to be affected by facial expression and tone of voice. The difference, therefore, between what the patient says and what the observer thinks, is not clear cut. The question really is whether the observer should try not to be influenced by subjective impressions, and attempt as far as possible to record the unmodified statement of the patient, or whether he should deliberately allow his clinical judgment and experience to colour his impressions. Some patients try to make light of their problems while others certainly appear to exaggerate their symptoms. It is what the patient feels that matters and it is only this that can give a measure of pain relief; but whether the patient is able or willing to describe this without help is a different matter. Many experienced physicians who have treated much pain in malignant disease come to rely upon the patient's face as much as anything, for it is here that true relief can often be seen (Maher 1975).

In many studies provision is made for the recording of both the patient's statement about pain and the observer's opinion. The differences are often not great, for the reasons already suggested, and the conclusions drawn from these supposedly separate assessments will not be significantly at variance. There is some evidence that the sensitivity of a study may be increased, at least in regard to the ability to distinguish an active drug from a placebo, if the observer's opinions are used (Parkhouse & Holmes 1963); but there is also evidence that this depends on who the observer is.

Apart from the possibility of slipshod work, or even deliberate invention of data, observers differ in their ability to assess pain and relief (Figs. 6.2 and 6.3). There is also the question of the consistency of one observer's judgments as time goes by. This was one of the principal advantages claimed for the use of an observer: the fact that, although patients may vary greatly, they will at least all be assessed by the same person. There is no doubt that this has important advantages over allowing a number of different people, for example the normal ward staff, to make assessments on the various patients included in a trial. However, as an observer grows older and more experienced, his assessments might change in character, and he may consciously or unconsciously alter his criteria even during the course of a single study. No rigorous studies have been made, although some observers in the United States have been carrying out this work for many years in an apparently stable manner, and have become valued members of the clinical teams concerned.

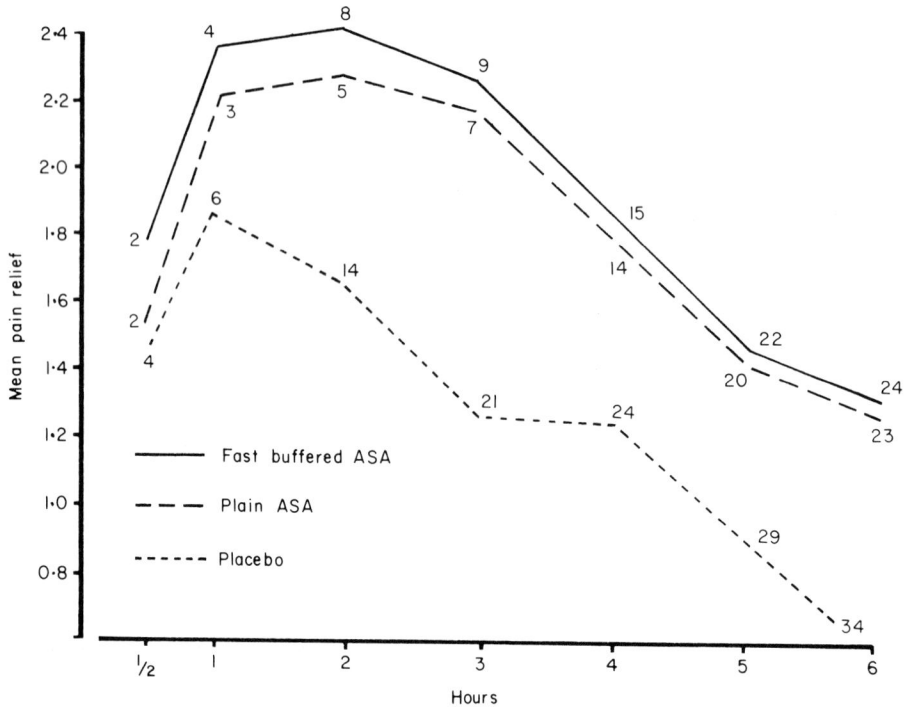

Figs. 6.2 and 6.3. Mean Pain Relief Scores in groups of patients at various times after oral administration of the drugs indicated. An identical study was carried out simultaneously in two hospitals, by two different nurse-observers. In hospital A (Fig. 6.2) a clear distinction is shown between aspirin and placebo, and the curves for the two aspirin preparations (in the same dosage) are virtually identical. In hospital B (Fig. 6.3) it is impossible to distinguish the placebo from the active drugs. The numbers on the curves indicate how many patients in each treatment group had already received a further drug for pain at the time interval shown. The total numbers of patients in the groups were, Fig. 6.2: 45 for the aspirin groups and 46 for the placebo; Fig. 6.3: 42 for the fast-buffered aspirin, 37 for normal aspirin and 39 for the placebo. (Originally published *C. M. A. Journal* **100**: 1057–58.)

3. Introspection and memory

Many philosophers and psychologists have debated the problem of trying immediately to describe sensations. William James in 1890 wrote:

'No subjective state, whilst present, is its own object; its object is

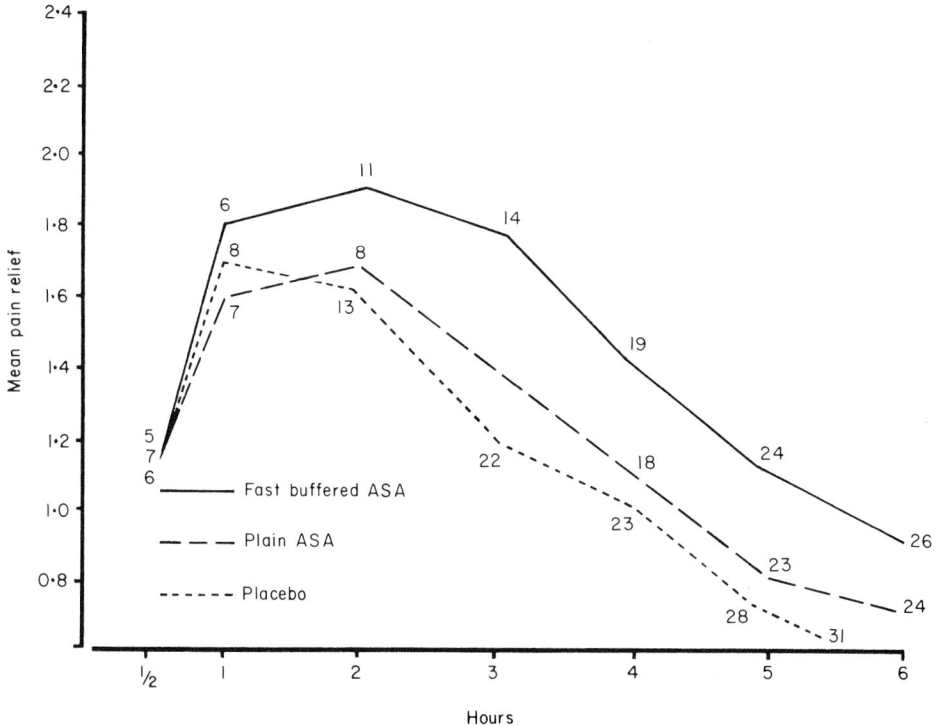

Fig. 6.3.

always something else. There are, it is true, cases in which we appear to be naming our present feeling, and so to be experiencing and observing the same inner fact at a single stroke, as when we say "I feel tired", "I am angry", etc. But these are illusory, and a little attention unmasks the illusion. The present conscious state, when I say "I feel tired", is not the direct state of tire; when I say "I feel angry", it is not the direct state of anger. It is the state of *saying-I-feel-tired*, of *saying-I-feel-angry*,—entirely different matters, so different that the fatigue and anger apparently included in them are considerable modifications of the fatigue and anger directly felt the previous instant. The act of naming them has momentarily detracted from their force.'

Much the same applies to pain. The alternative to seeking an instantaneous description of a painful experience is somewhat akin to what Wordsworth called emotion recollected in tranquility. For example, when a patient is asked which of two treatments was 'better' for his pain he is required to think back, and in some circumstances this undoubtedly creates problems. Similarly, if an observer asks at intervals how much 'better' the pain is, if at all, the patient may have difficulty in recalling exactly what he felt like before the test drug was given. In the extreme case of a patient recovering from an anaesthetic, the giving of a post-operative analgesic may not be remembered at all, although the pain that led to its administration was apparently unpleasant enough to cause extreme restlessness and vociferous pleas for relief.

The necessity for the patient to make mental comparisons between his feelings at various times is avoided by asking him on each occasion merely how he feels 'now'. This is what happens when a pain chart is provided, if it is properly used, and the same may be done by an observer. Any comparison, for example the subtraction of one pain score from another to give a measure of relief, can then be carried out independently of the patient.

In short-term studies where the point in question is the relative effectiveness of single doses of different drugs, the speed of onset or the duration of action, there are usually advantages in eliciting immediate assessment of pain 'now', particularly in circumstances where other drug effects or external events may interfere with the patient's recollection. In long-term studies or for more general conclusions about pain relief there may be advantages in asking the patient to make his own comparative estimates, either of the situation before and after treatment or of the value of alternative drugs.

It must be accepted that, however much the observer or even the patient himself may seek to capture the quintessence of the experience as it occurs, there is a difference between feeling a particular kind of pain and attempting to describe or record the feeling of it. It is equally true that, whatever shortcomings memory may have, and however 'inaccurate' retrospective impressions may be, there can be much usefulness in thinking back calmly over a sequence of events. No method of pain study is perfect; none even approaches the ideal. The resulting data are always a crude parody of the infinitely varied shades of human experience. Indeed, it is a sad comment on the inadequacy of our techniques that the most detailed and painstakingly recorded comments, when given by patients or observers, although interesting in themselves, are altogether too subtle and refined to be of any value in the processes of statistical analysis.

4. Signal detection theory

The possible application of Signal Detection Theory, or Sensory Decision Theory, to the evaluation of clinical pain and its relief has recently been discussed (Chapman 1974, Patton 1974). The theory arises from sophisticated studies in experimental psychology, concerned with the probability of detecting a given 'signal', against a background of neurophysiological activity. At the lowest limits of perception, the probability of a subject being correct in stating that a specific stimulus has been applied is a matter for statistical analysis. In the case of a painful stimulus, it is clear that if drug therapy or other methods of relief were to reduce the gap between 'background' and 'background plus signal', the probability of correctly recognizing the stimulus would be reduced. It is also suggested that the technique should be able to provide a measure of the subject's sensitivity to stimuli and, independently, of his bias towards describing such stimuli as painful (Clark 1974). The perceptive and reactive elements in pain reporting would thus be separated.

Signal Detection Theory offers potential advantages over the simple measurement of pain threshold, which has not proved to be of great value clinically. However, the application of Signal Detection Theory to assessment of pain modulation should not be accepted uncritically (Rollman 1976) and it has been pointed out (Taub 1974) that in the great majority of clinical situations the patient suffering from pain does not consciously wait upon his stimulus, does not make a decision in the true sense, and is concerned with 'signals' far above the threshold level.

5. Objective indices

Although pain is a subjective experience it may produce observable and even measurable effects. Facial expression, tone of voice, posture and gesture have already been mentioned in relation to the formation of an observer's impression. Autonomic concomitants such as sweating and pallor may be seen; changes in cutaneous electrical resistance may be measured. Preoccupation with pain distracts the patient's attention from other things, and measures of this can be devised; it has been suggested, for example, that two-point discrimination may vary with pain severity for this reason (Batterman 1963).

When the performance of a specified task is painful, this clearly provides the basis for a form of measurement. The most obvious example, perhaps, is the range of movement of a painful joint. In evaluating pain relief in arthritis, ranges of movement can be measured as angles, thus giving a numerical form to the data. Other examples of objective tests may come to mind, but the most important is the measurement of vital capacity as an index of pain after abdominal surgery.

It has long been acknowledged that the performance of a vital capacity measurement gives a mixture of information about the state of the lungs and about the patient's willingness to make the necessary effort. Overholt, in 1930, measured the vital capacity of 10 patients before upper abdominal surgery and noted a slight fall after giving 10 mg. of morphine. He then made the same measurements on the same patients after surgery, and repeated the same dose of morphine. The post-operative vital capacity was reduced to less than a third of the pre-operative average, and morphine improved it. This interesting early example of a controlled trial provided a convincing demonstration of the importance of pain in limiting deep breathing when the abdominal muscles have been interfered with, and of the need for adequate post-operative pain relief if chest complications are to be avoided. Subsequently, both vital capacity and peak expiratory flow measurements have been used as measures of pain and its relief in these circumstances (Bromage 1955, Parkhouse & Holmes 1963). As clinical tests they have the added advantage that their performance obliges the patient to do what is good for him.

The discussion of detail in regard to objective indices of pain is a specialised matter. Two principles, however, are of general importance. Firstly, a good score may mean less pain or more willingness to bear it.There is no escape from the compounding of pain and personality, but at least each patient serves as his own control when performing an objective test before and at intervals after treatment. Secondly, whenever a numerical measurement of performance is made in this context, it is merely an indication of something different—namely, pain. It is perhaps reassuring to the investigator to have a set of measured angles of movement or volumes of expired gas, rather than a set of subjective impressions of pain severity. The temptation is to apply statistics uncritically but the numbers are only a guide to what is happening in the mind; the pain behind the test is no more and no less linear in its progression and no more or less amenable to arithmetical manipulation than it was before.

6. Composite indices

In many situations it is obviously possible to obtain more than one guide to the patient's progress. Some investigators have deliberately used both subjective and objective assessment of pain in the hope that one might prove more sensitive than the other, or give additional information. There are dangers in this if the patient is subjected to too much attention, not all of which may be either welcome or in his best interests, and if there is any possibility of one evaluation interacting with or influencing the other.

Sometimes, as in chronic arthritis, pain has different qualities and effects which it would be as well to study separately. Pain at rest, for example, may respond to treatment differently from pain which limits movement. Also, pain relief in itself may be only one element in the overall picture of improvement. Whether morning stiffness can be evaluated separately from pain, or whether it is better regarded as a particular type of pain, is a case in point. Numerous studies have resulted in the compilation of data on several separate criteria—morning stiffness, pain at rest, range of movement of specified joints, daily demand for analgesics, and others. Each set of data may be analysed separately; alternatively, a composite index may be made up in which each factor is weighted according to the investigator's view of its importance. In some cases such composite indices are undoubtedly useful, but the investigator employs them at his peril. He must be prepared to face the judgment of his colleagues and of the statisticians; it is best, therefore, to show the individual criteria, at least in summary, so that the reader can draw his own conclusions or make up a different index for comparative purposes. Mainland (1964) provides an interesting and readily intelligible discussion of composite indices.

Principles and problems of statistical interpretation

There is a close interdependence between the design of a clinical experiment, the tactics of its conduct and the analysis of its results. No trial should be conceived without some inkling of how the data are to be handled. It is essential to foresee the problems that particular kinds of data will create for statistical analysis; otherwise much time and money may be wasted in carrying out a study that is foredoomed to be inconclusive. An hour spent with a statistician during the planning of a trial can save days of frustration at its end.

Statisticians are sometimes blamed for the intricacy and sophistication of the techniques they apply. Although such comment may occasionally be justified, there are two things to be said. Firstly, the effort expended on statistical analysis is insignificant compared to the labour of obtaining the data that are to be analysed. When a clinician has taken meticulous care to carry out a complex study, and when this has involved the voluntary cooperation of sick people as subjects, any reputable statistician will feel it incumbent upon him to miss nothing in the data that may be of value or interest. Secondly, what is done by the statistician is all too often a rescue operation in which special and perhaps laborious methods are needed to compensate for faults in planning or execution. Statisticians are well aware of the inherent variability of biological data, and many are conversant with the pitfalls and difficulties of clinical investigation; they are usually as keen as the clinician himself should be to keep things as simple as possible.

Scales and steps

The use of numbers is based primarily upon counting of objects. If two chairs are brought into a room which already contains one chair, there will be a total of three chairs in the room. Removing two would leave one; doubling the number would make six and squaring it, nine. This says nothing at all about the sizes, shapes and weights of the chairs, which may all be different; it refers merely to the number, upon which any legitimate mathematical operation can be applied. Two plus one is, by definition, exactly three and never anything else.

If we wish to study the heaviness or heights of the chairs we need to apply our counting to recognized units of weight or length. Providing the units are standardized we can then add up the measurements and calculate an average weight or length. This is possible because again, two kilograms plus one kilogram is exactly three kilograms and never anything else.

It is important to realize that there are some situations in which we have enough information to make truly quantitative assessments of the degree or extent of a given quality, such as weight, and other situations in which all that can be done is to enumerate objects or people. This fundamental difference is reflected in the availability of different types of statistical analysis.

When arbitrary 'steps' are used to define degrees of pain, such as mild, moderate and severe it has to be remembered that these steps are not necessarily equal. Nor are they necessarily the same for different individuals; a change from moderate to slight pain may seem unimportant to one patient compared to a change from severe pain to moderate pain; but for another patient it might make all the difference (Lasagna 1960). The same considerations apply to movement along an arbitrary scale or chart. It is simple to use the digits 1, 2 and 3 to signify mild, moderate and severe, and hence derive average 'pain scores' for groups of patients, with standard errors, but the soundness of the mathematical basis for this is clearly very much open to question. In practice, it yields usable results which are unlikely to be seriously misleading, but much thought has been given to ways of avoiding the 'equal step' problem.

A further problem with step-wise descriptions of pain intensity is that patients who begin with only mild or moderate pain cannot possibly show, in the pseudo-numerical terms of these steps, as much relief as those patients who begin with severe pain. This difficulty has worried a number of investigators (e.g. Parkhouse & Hallinon 1967), because in subjective terms it is apparent that relief of moderate pain may be just as valuable to the sufferer as relief from severe pain, and it seems important to be able to make this point. The clinical evaluation by this means of drugs specifically intended to relieve mild pain is made very difficult by the fact that the maximum possible improvement is only very small. The problem can be overcome to some extent by seeking an assessment from the patient of relief, as opposed to pain. Then the patient has the opportunity of rating his relief highly even when his original pain was not severe. Difficulties of statistical analysis are not eased, and degrees of relief do not step any more equally than those of pain.

Significance tests

Bearing in mind the above considerations, groups of patients may be compared in several ways.

Firstly, an arbitrary criterion can be selected and the number of patients in each group who meet the criterion can be counted. This is the simplest form of comparison. It may be based on an 'all or none' distinction between success of treatment and failure—e.g. those patients obtaining relief of pain and those not relieved; alternatively, a number of grades of relief may be recognised. In either case a χ^2 test

can be applied and a great deal of information can be obtained without making potentially dubious assumptions about the quantitative
nature of the data. An excellent account of the uses of the χ^2 test in
these situations is given by Maxwell (1961).

Secondly, the patients studied can be placed in order of rank
according to the criterion of interest, for example the patients with
the greatest pain relief at the top of the list and those with least relief
at the bottom. If two alternative analgesics were used, it is then
possible to see if most of the patients who received one of the drugs lie
at the top of the table or if the distribution is even. A number of
so-called non-parametric statistical tests are based on this kind of
ranking procedure; they enable the observed distribution to be
compared with the complete lack of order that would be expected on
the 'null hypothesis' that neither drug was better than the other. As
with other significance tests the probability of a difference as large as
that observed occurring simply by chance is used as a guide to the
meaningfulness of the findings. Non-parametric tests of this type
avoid the 'equal step' problem; the data are merely placed in order of
magnitude and nothing is said or assumed about the size of the step
from one entry in the list to the next. Non-parametric tests are also
sometimes described as 'distribution free', since they do not depend
for their validity on the individual items of data being normally distributed, i.e. following a Gaussian distribution. A considerable range
of non-parametric tests and a useful introduction to their use is given
by Siegel (1956).

Thirdly, groups of patients can be compared by the traditional
method of taking the average 'score' for those in each group and
examining, by means of the standard deviation or the standard error
of the mean, the closeness with which the individual scores in each
group are gathered about the group mean. The distance between the
means for the groups can then be looked at in relation to this. This is
the basis of Student's t-test. Use of the test does raise the equal-step
problem, already discussed. It is a test intended for normally distributed data and its relevance to clinical pain studies might be
questioned; there is no reason, for example, why scores for pain relief
should be normally distributed about a mean and they certainly
would not be expected to be so distributed about zero, i.e. for patients
to be equally likely to get worse or better. In fact, the t-test is a
'robust' test and departures from the Gaussian distribution do not
have a disastrous effect (Boneau 1960); for theoretical reasons it is

more important to the t-test for the means of different samples from a population to be normally distributed than for the individual data to follow this pattern.

When significance tests are used on clinical data it is usually felt that the result can be regarded as 'statistically significant' if a difference as large as that observed would not be likely to occur purely by chance more often than once in 20 trials (i.e. a P value of 1 in 20, or 0·05). Since this argument applies to each test, a problem can arise when multiple t-tests are performed. If three drugs A, B and C are compared with a placebo, D, it is possible to carry out t-tests comparing A with B, A with C, A with D, B with C, B with D, and C with D. Each of these tests can be applied to more than one assessment, for instance the patients' estimates of pain and the observer's estimates of relief. If the assessments have been made at hourly intervals, t-test comparisons can be made of the scores at each hour, and of the total scores. Altogether, therefore, 84 t-tests might be carried out. This is something of a magnifico ad absurdum, but it would not be surprising if, by sheer chance, one or more of the results appeared to be 'statistically significant'. On the other hand it may not be easy to choose in advance which comparisons it is most profitable to make. This problem of multiple comparisons can be overcome by using specially designed statistical tests such as Duncan's (1955) multiple range test or an appropriate extension (Kramer 1956). With these tests it is possible to show, by underlining, which comparisons do not show statistically significant differences at the 5 per cent or any other chosen level: e.g.

$$\underline{A \qquad \underline{B \qquad C}} \qquad D$$

indicates that the differences between B and B and between B and C were not significant but the other differences (A/C, A/D, B/D, C/D) were significant.

Sequential statistical analysis is usually based on preferences or simple yes/no decisions. For example each point may be plotted according to which of two analgesics (given to the same patient or to two successive patients in the trial) yielded a better result. This better result might be a higher score for relief, a subjectively expressed preference or some other indication of effect; but it is not a quantitative difference and the size of the 'step' between the effects of the two drugs does not enter into any calculation. Some theoretical difficulties are thus avoided, although if the differences between drugs are in fact very large the technique will clearly be relatively insensitive. If it is thought to be desirable a sequential *t*-test can in fact be carried out, using the actual quantitative difference within in each pair of observations (Armitage 1960).

Analysis of variance

When observations are compared it will be obvious that they differ, one from another, for various reasons. The patients may be different, the effects of the drugs may be different, the underlying pain may have changed and there may be many other possible influences. The purpose of analysis of variance is to separate these factors and discover how much of the variation between individuals, or treatment groups is due to each. It is thus a very powerful statistical tool.

Although the mathematics are often fairly complex, the principle can be illustrated by a simple example. Suppose two patients are given two drugs, *A* and *B*, in succession, but in one case *A* followed *B* and in the other case *B* followed by *A*. A series of possibilities can be envisaged:

1. If the drugs are equal in their effect, and all other factors are equal, the responses of both patients to both drugs will be the same. Let us assume this is a response of 5 units. The result can be shown thus:

	Patient receiving	Response to 1st dose	Response to 2nd dose	1st dose response + 2nd dose response	1st dose response − 2nd dose response
Patient 1	*A* *B*	5	5	10	0
Patient 2	*B* *A*	5	5	10	0

2. If the first patient shows a better response to drugs in general than the second patient (variation between patients) his relief score will be higher than Patient *B*'s for both doses:

Patient 1	*A* *B*	6	6	12	0
Patient 2	*B* *A*	5	5	10	0

3. If drug *A* is better than drug *B* (variation between drugs) the response to drug *A* will be higher for both patients:

| Patient 1 | A | B | 6 | 4 | 10 | +2 |
| Patient 2 | B | A | 4 | 6 | 10 | −2 |

4. If the pain has improved during the study, so that the second dose always appears more effective (variation with time) each patient, irrespective of the order in which the drugs were given, will show a better response to the second dose:

| Patient 1 | A | B | 5 | 6 | 11 | −1 |
| Patient 2 | B | A | 5 | 6 | 11 | −1 |

5. If the effect of drug A is sufficiently persistent to influence a subsequent drug administration, while the effect of drug B is not (variation with order of administration) the response to the second dose will be higher when drug A has been given first, but not after drug B:

| Patient 1 | A | B | 5 | 6 | 11 | −1 |
| Patient 2 | B | A | 5 | 5 | 10 | 0 |

All possible combinations of these circumstances, and others, could now be tested. By inspection of the last two columns it will become clear that each yields a distinctive pattern. Application of the proper mathematical techniques makes it possible to see not only which sources of variation are operative but also to what extent each contributes to the total scatter of the individual scores.

Combining of data

There are superficial attractions in the idea of combining data from two or more studies in order to assemble a greater mass of information for statistical analysis. Such studies may be carried out simultaneously in different hospitals or in different cities (Bellville *et al.* 1968 a, b). The recording of data can be standardized (Parkhouse 1967) and the techniques and criteria for assessment and scoring can be agreed beforehand. Indeed, the nurse-observers or whoever will make the subjective assessments may work together for an initial trial period or may originate from the same training centre. The natural differences in exuberance between observers' scoring can if necessary be compensated for by a process akin to 'scaling up' or 'scaling down', so that the range of response is uniform for all the data; acceptable statistical techniques are available for this (e.g. RIDIT analysis, Bross 1958).

It seems an inescapable fact that some observers, in some hospitals, obtain better discrimination between drugs than others. Insofar as this is the important thing, the only effect of pooling data from more than one study will be to adulterate valuable information. If the aim is to achieve maximum efficiency, in the sense of learning about clinically significant differences in the primary effect of drugs with the least delay and expense, there is therefore nothing to be gained by combining data from several studies. If it is felt to be more important to know how the different drugs appear in a variety of clinical circumstances, and in different people's hands, then more than one study is clearly needed, and each must be separately analysed. Combining of the data may then give some supplementary information of a general kind, as may be had from composite indices. Finally, the gathering up of as much data as possible, from a number of controlled trials or from surveys, will reveal occasional phenomena that may be of consequence, including side effects.

Conclusion

The controlled clinical trial has developed into a valuable and effective means of finding out about drugs. In some respects this may be said less enthusiastically about analgesics than some other drugs, but in general the statement is valid.

What a controlled trial cannot be expected to achieve is fairly clear: it will not answer badly formulated questions precisely and it will not answer multiple questions with equal facility. A small trial will not uncover rare events and statistical analysis will not explain unusual cases (although it may draw attention to them). It is most of all necessary to recall that individual patients vary, in their complaint and in response to its attempted relief. In post-operative pain, for example, this variation has been studied and reported (Papper *et al.* 1952, Parkhouse *et al.* 1961). It remains true, therefore, that the treatment of each separate patient is a different matter from the analysis of the average response of a group. Controlled trials provide a yardstick for the introduction of new drugs and are of help in deciding contentious issues about certain specific effects; they are not necessarily an infallible guide to the clinical management of each patient.

Appendix 1 · Some Statistical Examples

The general principles of statistical analysis, and the purpose of carrying out significance tests, will be apparent from the foregoing chapter. By way of amplification, the following section is intended to help the reader by providing simple examples of some of the actual ways in which data from a controlled trial of analgesic drugs might be handled statistically. The artificial data used in this section conveniently exemplify a number of the problems that may arise in the interpretation and analysis of real data. For purposes of illustration it is useful to take the same data and handle them in different ways; this is not intended to imply, however, that in reality all the statistical methods shown would be equally applicable to the same set of data. In fact, the orthodox view would be that the data given in this section are really only suitable for non-parametric analysis. It should also be emphasized that no attempt is made here to enter into detailed theoretical considerations.

A point that may usefully be clarified at the outset is the distinction between 'one-tailed' and 'two-tailed' tests. In some circumstances there is only one direction in which events can possibly move. A study of changes in the temperature of a pan of water during the constant application of heat might show whether or not it is possible to demonstrate a statistically significant rise in temperature over a given short period of time. The question of observing a fall in temperature does not arise, since the possibility does not exist. In such a situation one would be concerned with the probability of observing a change in one direction only and a 'one tailed' test would be appropriate. In clinical practice such situations almost never arise. When a patient is given an analgesic, there is no guarantee that his pain will not actually get worse after the drug has been given, and all clinicians know that this sometimes happens. Likewise, when an active drug is compared with a placebo the investigator may occasionally be faced with the embarrassment of a result which appears to show a statistically significant difference in favour of the placebo. Certainly, when two active drugs are to be compared, there is normally no sure way of knowing in advance which is likely to be the better. In these circumstances the probability of observing a significant difference between the drugs must be taken to mean the combined probabilities of finding that *A* is better than *B* and of finding that *B* is better than *A*. In relation to the normal distribution, the difference may occur either in the upper 'tail' of the curve or in the lower 'tail'; hence in these situations a 'two tailed' test is appropriate. Some further reference to this point occurs in relation to the individual tests described below.

Results of an imaginary trial

Suppose that two analgesics, *A* and *B*, have both been given to 20 patients. The trial has been carried out 'double blind', and ran-

Table A.1.

	First Dose		Second Dose		
Patient	Drug	Relief Score	Drug	Relief Score	Preference
1	*B*	3	*A*	2	*B*
2	*B*	2	*A*	2	=
3	*A*	1	*B*	2	*B*
4	*A*	2	*B*	3	*B*
5	*A*	0	*B*	1	*B*
6	*B*	2	*A*	3	*A*
7	*B*	3	*A*	0	*B*
8	*B*	1	*A*	1	=
9	*A*	0	*B*	3	*B*
10	*B*	2	*A*	2	=
11	*A*	1	*B*	3	*B*
12	*A*	1	*B*	2	*B*
13	*A*	2	*B*	1	*A*
14	*B*	3	*A*	2	*B*
15	*B*	1	*A*	0	*B*
16	*A*	0	*B*	3	*B*
17	*B*	3	*A*	1	*B*
18	*A*	3	*B*	3	=
19	*A*	0	*B*	2	*B*
20	*B*	3	*A*	1	*B*

domized in order to ensure that half the patients received A as a first dose and B as a second dose, and the other half received the drugs in the opposite order; whether any individual patient received A or B first was also decided by random allocation. The results of treatment were scored in terms of the pain relief obtained, according to the following scale: $0 =$ No Relief, $1 =$ Poor Relief, $2 =$ Moderate Relief, $3 =$ Good Relief.

The results turned out as shown in Table A.1.

Chi-squared test

A simple way of looking at the above results, which has the advantages described in the text of Chapter 6, is to decide on a criterion which defines 'relief of pain'. Let us suppose that a score of 0 or 1 means that the patient was not relieved, while a score of 2 or 3 means that he obtained relief.

It is then possible to draw up a table showing how many of the patients were relieved, or not relieved, after receiving each of the drugs (Table A.2).

For the purposes of this table all scores have been included, regardless of whether they relate to first or second doses. The table is the simplest form of Chi-squared table, consisting of two rows and two columns and hence known as a 2×2 table.

It is obvious from inspection of the table that the number of patients relieved by drug B, according to the agreed criterion, was much higher than the number relieved by A, in fact twice as many. This agrees with the impression drawn from the last column of Table A.1, which shows that 14 of the 20 patients 'preferred' B to A, in other words obtained a better relief score from B, while only 2 preferred A to B. On common-sense grounds we therefore have fairly good reason for supposing that B was a more effective analgesic, in this particular trial, than A.

Table A.2

Drug	Not Relieved	Relieved	Total
A	12	8	20
B	4	16	20
Total	16	24	40

Pain score 0 or 1 = not relieved; pain score 2 or 3 = relieved.

Table A.3.

Drug	Relieved	Not Relieved	Total
A	a	b	$a + b$
B	c	d	$c + d$
Total	$a + c$	$b + d$	$a + b + c + d$ $(= N)$

To assess whether the difference between A and B is 'statistically significant' the value of Chi-squared can be calculated from the figures in the table, which may be represented symbolically as shown in Table A.3.

$$\chi^2 = \frac{(ad - bc - N/2)^2 \times (N)}{(a + b) \times (c + d) \times (a + c) \times (b + d)}$$

This formula incorporates Yates' Correction (the subtraction of half the grand total in the first bracket of the numerator) which greatly improves the agreement between the Chi-squared test and exact tests of significance.*

For the data that we have,

$$\chi^2 = \frac{(12 \times 16 - 8 \times 4 - 20)^2 \times 40}{20 \times 20 \times 16 \times 24}$$

$$= \frac{(160 - 20)^2 \times 40}{20 \times 20 \times 16 \times 24}$$

$$= 5 \cdot 104$$

We now consult a table of Chi-squared values, selecting the appropriate number of 'degrees of freedom'. The number of 'degrees of freedom' is determined by the number of classes among the results which could be assigned arbitrarily while still maintaining the same totals and sub-totals. In the present case, we know that a total of 20 patients received drug A, so if 12 of these were not relieved the number 'relieved' must be 8 and could not be altered to anything else. Likewise, since the total number of patients 'not relieved' was 16,

* Yates' Correction is known as a 'correction for continuity' since it allows for the fact that, while the Chi-squared distribution is a continuous distribution, the actual data represent a non-continuous or binomial type of distribution (see later).

then if 12 of these received drug *A* the number who received drug *B* must have been 4. Thus, once any one of the 4 values *a*, *b*, *c*, *d* has been fixed the others are also determined, and there is therefore only one 'degree of freedom'. This will, of course, apply to every 2 × 2 table.

From the Chi-squared table, for one degree of freedom, we find

$$0.05 > P > 0.01$$

This means that the probability (*P*) of the amount of difference that we observed between *A* and *B* occurring purely by chance, rather than as a result of any actual difference between the two drugs, is less than 0.05 but greater than 0.01—in other words, less than a 1 in 20 chance but more than a 1 in 100 chance. According to the conventional standards applied to controlled clinical trials, we would therefore regard the result as 'statistically significant'.

There are reservations about the use of the Chi-squared test for small numbers of cases. The usual convention is that the expected number in any one cell should not be less than 5. It is important to note that this is the 'expected' number. The actual number of patients not relieved after drug *B* is only 4, but since a total of 16 out of 40 patients were not relieved, and 20 patients received each drug, we would have expected that if *A* and *B* were equally likely to leave a patient unrelieved the number of patients in this cell would have been 8 (exactly half the total number of unrelieved patients). Since this smallest 'expected' cell content is over 5, use of the Chi-squared test is justified.

The formula given above is a shorthand calculation specifically applicable to 2 × 2 tables. The whole principle of the Chi-squared test depends upon examining the size of the difference between *observed* numbers in each class and the numbers that would be *expected* on the 'null hypothesis' that there is no difference between the treatments.

INTERACTIONS AND PARTITIONING

An important consideration with regard to the Chi-squared test is whether or not there is any interaction between the groups of cases studied. Such interactions may occur in a number of ways.

From the imaginary results used here, it is fairly obvious that *B* is a better drug than *A*. Not only does this emerge from the individual relief scores, but there is also a suggestion that when *A* is given following *B* it produces a better result than when given first. This may well happen if one of the drugs in a trial has a powerful and long-lasting effect.

The results can be displayed as shown in Table A.4.a.

From this table it can be seen that the number of patients 'relieved' by *B* is exactly the same regardless of whether it is given as the first dose or the second dose, whereas with *A* 5 out of 10 patients were 'relieved' when the drug was given following *B*, compared to only 3 out of 10 when it did not follow *B*. To see whether the difference within the *A* results is significant, Chi-squared can be partitioned as a simple form of analysis of variance. For the purpose of this partitioning there is no point in subdividing the *B* results, since there is clearly no 'order effect' in the case of *B*. The above table can therefore be simplified into a 3 × 2 table in order to look separately at the difference between *A* 1st dose and *A* 2nd dose, and the difference between *A* (both doses) and *B* (Table A.4.b).

The method used for partitioning Chi-squared is explained in detail by Maxwell (1961).

Firstly, an overall test gives a Chi-squared value of 7·5 which, with two degrees of freedom, is significant at the level $P < 0.025$.

Table A.4.a.

	A 1st dose	*A* 2nd dose	*B* 1st dose	*B* 2nd dose	Total
Relieved	3	5	8	8	24
Not Relieved	7	5	2	2	16
Total	10	10	10	10	40

Table A.4.b.

	A 1st dose	*A* 2nd dose	*B*	Total
Relieved	3	5	16	24
Not Relieved	7	5	4	16
Total	10	10	20	40

Partitioning according to the formulae of Kimball, quoted by Maxwell (1961) yields the following:

$$A \text{ 1st dose compared to } A \text{ 2nd dose } \chi_1^2 = 0.8333$$

$$A \text{ (both doses) compared with } B \; \chi_2^2 = 6.6666$$

Each of these values has one degree of freedom, so that

$$\chi_1^2 \text{ not significant}$$

$$\chi_2^2 P < 0.01$$

(It should be noted that the sum of these two component values of Chi-squared equals 7·4999, i.e. the same as the overall Chi-squared value).

The unpaired *t*-test

In this section, and the following section on the paired *t*-test, the method of working closely follows that set out by Swinscow (1976).

For the *first dose* given to each patient, the relief scores obtained from *A* and *B* can be listed as follows, with the relevant calculations (Table A.5.).

The average (mean) relief score for *B* is clearly considerably higher than for *A*, and by calculating the Standard Deviation for each set of results we have an estimate of the spread about each of the means. Assuming that the results follow a normal distribution, we know that about 95% of the observations in each set will lie within 2 Standard Deviations on either side of the mean for the set. The results could be represented graphically (Fig. A.1) although it should be remembered that this illustration is based on a very small number of results and what we are really interested in are the true means and Standard Deviations of the 'population' as a whole: i.e., to return to the 'null hypothesis' principle, we wish to know whether, if we studied a very large number of cases, there would really be any difference between the means for *A* and *B* or whether all the results would form part of one single population.

The area up to 2 Standard Deviations above the mean for *A* has been hatched, and likewise the area up to 2 Standard Deviations below the mean for *B*. Inspection shows that, although the means are quite well separated, there is a considerable degree of overlap in the results. In other words, quite a number of the observations recorded

Appendix 1

Table A.5. Unpaired *t*-test.

		A	B
		1	3
		2	2
		0	2
		0	3
		1	1
		1	2
		2	3
		0	1
		3	3
		0	3
Sum	Σx	10	23
Mean	$\dfrac{\Sigma x}{n}$	1·00	2·30
Sum of squares	Σx^2	20	59
Squared sum	$(\Sigma x)^2$	100	529
Squared sum divided by no. of observations, n (10 for each drug)	$\dfrac{(\Sigma x)^2}{n}$	10·0	52·9
	$\Sigma x^2 - \dfrac{(\Sigma x)^2}{n}$	10·0*	6·1*
Estimate of variance (S.D. squared)	$\dfrac{\Sigma x^2 - (\Sigma x)^2/n}{n-1}$	1·111	0·678
Standard deviation		1·054	0·822

after *A* lie within the distribution *B* and could equally well have resulted from the administration of *B*. Furthermore, the variances, and hence the Standard Deviations, of the two samples are not the same; the *B* results are more closely grouped around the mean than the *A* results. In fact, the mean for *B* is almost exactly 2 Standard Deviations (of *B*) above the mean for *A*, but the same could not be said the other way round; the mean for *A* is considerably less than 2 Standard Deviations (of *A*) below the mean for *B*.

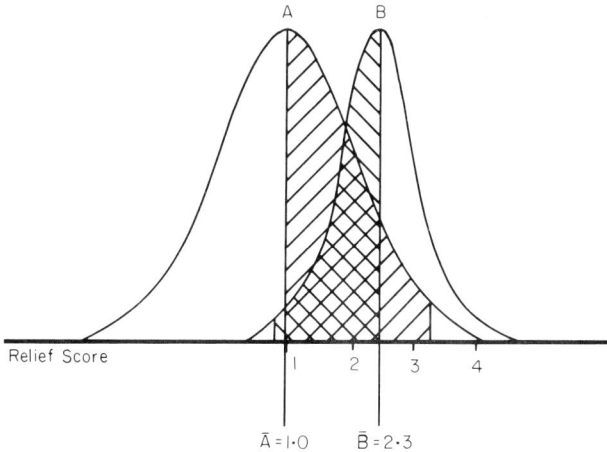

Fig. A.1. Graphical representation of the relief scores for drugs A and B.

We could form an impression of whether there is likely to be a 'statistically significant' difference by looking at the standard error of the difference between the means. This is calculated by taking each of the variances for A and B, as calculated above, dividing them by the number of observations in each group, adding the results together and taking the square root. The standard error of the difference is thus the square root of $0.111 + 0.0678$, which equals 0.423. Since the difference between means, 1.3, is about three times the standard error of the difference we can be fairly sure that this result would not arise by chance.

Before proceeding to a complete t-test it is advisable to confirm that the difference in variance of the two samples is not of significant proportions. This is because, theoretically, the t-test is based on the assumption that the two samples are both normally distributed and of equal variance. The F test can be used to calculate the variance ratio from the two samples, the procedure being described by Moroney (1951) and in other standard books. The procedure is as follows:

$$F = \frac{\text{estimate of variance for } A}{\text{estimate of variance for } B} = \frac{1.111}{0.678} = 1.639$$

Reference to the appropriate table (also given and explained by Moroney, 1951) shows that the result is below the critical value for F for the appropriate numbers of degrees of freedom, and that therefore the variances do not differ significantly.

To complete the calculation of the value of t, we use the results in Table A.5 marked by asterisks, which were derived from sums of squares and squared sums of observations in the table:

Variance of difference (Standard Error of difference squared)
$$\frac{10\cdot0 + 6\cdot1}{n_1 + n_2 - 2} = \frac{10\cdot0 + 6\cdot1}{10 + 10 - 2} = 0\cdot894$$

$$\text{S.E. of difference} = \sqrt{\left(\frac{0\cdot894}{10} + \frac{0\cdot894}{10}\right)} = 0\cdot423$$

(the same as derived above from the individual variances)

$$t = \frac{\text{difference of means}}{\text{S.E. of difference}} = \frac{2\cdot3 - 1\cdot0}{0\cdot423} = 3\cdot073$$

The appropriate number of degrees of freedom is, once again, the number of observations that could be given arbitrarily assigned values, while still retaining the same sub-totals and grand total. It is clear that for A nine of the ten observations could be given any arbitrary value, but this would determine what the tenth value had to be in order to give the correct total of 10; likewise any nine of the B results could be arbitrarily assigned as long as the tenth observation made the total 23. Thus, the total number of degrees of freedom is 18, the same as the denominator used in calculating the variance of the difference. Reference to the appropriate table of t, for 18 degrees of freedom, shows that $0\cdot01 > P > 0\cdot002$.

The paired t-test

Since each patient was treated with each drug, it is possible to look at the differences in the relief scores obtained from A and B for each case (Table A.6.). This, of course, involves using the data for both first doses and second doses, but it enables a t-test to be carried out on

Table A.6.

Differences ($A-B$)									
-1	0	-1	-1	-1	$+1$	-3	0	-3	0
-2	-1	$+1$	-1	-1	-3	-2	0	-2	-2

pairs of observations. This simplifies the arithmetic and leads to increased sensitivity.

The method of working is given below, following the description given by Swinscow (1976).

$$\text{sum of differences } \Sigma d = -22$$

$$\text{mean of differences } \bar{d} = -1\cdot10$$

$$\text{sum of differences squared } \Sigma d^2 = 52$$

$$\text{squared sum of differences } (\Sigma d)^2 = 484$$

$$\frac{(\Sigma d)^2}{n} = 24\cdot2$$

$$\Sigma d^2 - \frac{(\Sigma d)^2}{n} = 27\cdot8$$

$$\frac{\Sigma d^2 - (\Sigma d)^2/n}{n-1} = 1\cdot463$$

$$\frac{SD^2}{n} = 0\cdot0731$$

$$\sqrt{\frac{SD^2}{n}} = 0\cdot2704$$

The final figure arrived at above, $0\cdot2704$, is the standard error of the mean of the differences. The mean of the differences, $1\cdot10$, is divided by this in order to derive t:

$$t = \frac{1\cdot10}{0\cdot2704}$$

In this case there are 19 degrees of freedom (one less than the total number of differences) and reference to the appropriate table shows that

$$P < 0\cdot001$$

This is a 'highly significant' result which demonstrates that by using paired data, for both first and second doses, a good deal more sensitivity is achieved than by performing an unpaired t-test on first doses alone, as above.

A non-parametric test

The data we have available from this imaginary trial are ordinal: they indicate degrees of relief which can be arranged in order of magnitude from 0 to 3, but they do not represent actual measurements against any universally acknowledged scale. There is thus legitimate concern about the 'equal step problem' referred to in the previous chapter. It is also clear that the data collected may not be normally distributed. These are sound reasons for preferring the use of a non-parametric test.

An example would be the Wilcoxon Rank Sum Test, the details of which can be found in standard books such as Siegel (1956). A simple illustration is given by Swinscow (1976).

The test is based on putting the differences in observed scores for A and B, for the individual patients, in order of magnitude, i.e. ranking them from the largest to the smallest. The first column that is required, therefore, is exactly the same as the one used for the Paired *t*-test above, showing the differences between A and B scores in each case. The remainder of the procedure is shown to the right of this column (Table A.7).

Where the score for A and B is identical (0 difference) no rank is assigned. All differences of 1 are ties and are therefore given the same rank. This is regardless of whether the difference is positive or negative. In Table A.7, there are 9 differences of 1 and these therefore collectively occupy the first 9 ranks (1–9) and are each given the average rank of 5·0. The 4 differences of 2 occupy jointly the rank positions from 10–13, and therefore each get the average rank of 11·5. The remaining 3 differences, which are differences of 3, occupy the remaining ranks from 14–16 and hence each receive an average rank of 15.

The next step in the procedure is to attach a positive or negative sign to each of the ranks derived as above, according to whether the originally observed difference is positive or negative. This is shown in the final column of Table A.7. The totals for the positive and for the negative signed ranks are next inspected, and whichever is the smaller is referred to the appropriate tables. In our example, the total of the signed ranks bearing a plus is obviously smaller than the total of the signed ranks bearing a minus. The positive total is $5 + 5 = 10$. Reference to the table given by Swinscow (1976), for 16 pairs of ranked observations, shows that a total of 19 would be significant at the 1 per

Table A.7. Wilcoxon Rank Sum Test.

Difference in Scores $(A - B)$	Rank	Signed Rank
− 1	5·0	− 5
0		
− 1	5·0	− 5
− 1	5·0	− 5
− 1	5·0	− 5
+ 1	5·0	+ 5
− 3	15·0	− 15
0		
− 3	15·0	− 15
0		
− 2	11·5	− 11·5
− 1	5·0	− 5
+ 1	5·0	+ 5
− 1	5·0	− 5
− 1	5·0	− 5
− 3	15·0	− 15
− 2	11·5	− 11·5
0		
− 2	11·5	− 11·5
− 2	11·5	− 11·5

cent level ($P = 0.01$) and therefore our total of 10, being considerably *below* this value, is highly significant. The number used in referring to the table is not the total number of pairs of observations but the number of *ranked* observations (i.e. not counting the zero differences between A and B).

It will be obvious that a great advantage of this type of test is the simplicity of the calculations. Our example is not a particularly good case for the application of this test, since there are a large number of ties. This does not, however, invalidate the conclusions since the existence of ties tends to reduce the sensitivity of the test: i.e. there is rather more chance of failing to demonstrate a significant difference when one actually exists.

Sequential analysis

A sequential design suitable for this type of trial is shown in Fig. A.2.

The figures on the horizontal axis are numbers of pairs of cases studied. Preferences are shown on the vertical axis; movement in an

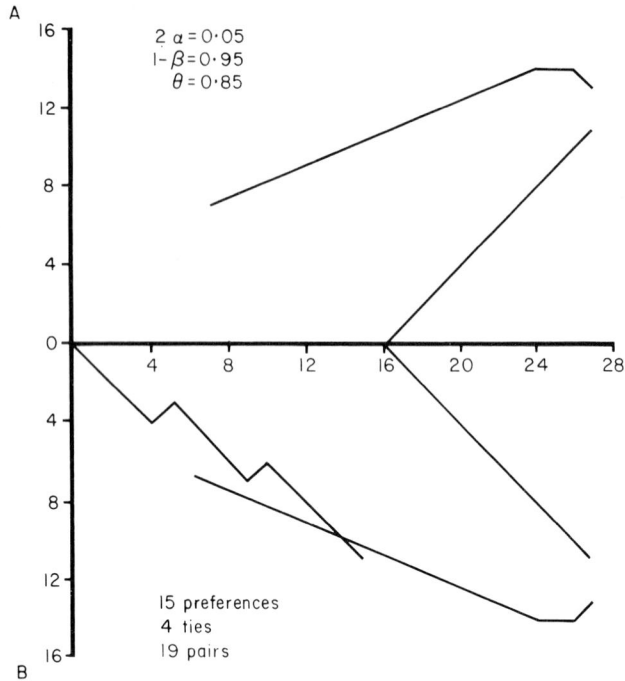

Fig. A.2. Sequential design for imaginary trial.

upward direction would denote that *A* was better than *B*, and downwards movement that *B* was better than *A*.

Details of relevant sequential methods are given by Armitage (1960), from whose book the design used for this illustration is selected. The boundaries of the design are arranged so that crossing of the upper boundary indicates that *A* has been shown to be superior to *B*, at a level of statistical significance previously decided upon, while crossing of the lower boundary indicates a corresponding decision in favour of *B*. The actual specifications for the design used are shown above the graph.

The designation '$2\alpha = 0.05$' is the probability of a 'type 1' error. This is the probability of wrongly rejecting the null hypothesis, that is falsely concluding that a significant difference exists. In practice, for there to be a significant difference between *A* and *B* there are clearly two possibilities—either that *A* is significantly better than *B* or that *B* is significantly better than *A*. These possibilities can be regarded as corresponding to the upper and lower 'tails' of the normal distribution (each probability being equal to α). Before the clinical trial is carried out we usually have no means of knowing which eventuality is more likely, and it is therefore better to take both possibilities into account: '2α' thus denotes the probability of being wrong in one direction (e.g. A better than B) plus the probability of being wrong in the other, and it is assumed that these probabilities are equal. In the terminology that we have become accustomed to, this is equivalent to the 'level of significance' at which the difference will be detected; if the boundary of the sequential design is drawn according to the specification for $2\alpha = 0.05$ this means that when the boundary is crossed the difference between A and B will be significant at the 0.05 level ($P = 0.05$)*. The designation 'β' is equal to the probability of the opposite kind of error ('type 2' error)—the risk of failing to detect a statistically significant difference when one exists. How likely it is that a true difference between A and B will be detected naturally depends on how large the difference between A and B actually is. The value for θ in the sequential diagram indicates the probability of preferring one drug to the other, and the term '$1 - \beta$' is an indication of the 'power' of the test.

In practice, the choice of a diagram is usually a compromize between the amount of 'power' or sensitivity that is required and the amount of data that is likely to be available. A design which gives a very high probability of detecting a very small difference between two drugs, at a high level of statistical significance (e.g. $P < 0.001$) will require a very large number of comparisons before the boundary can possibly be crossed. Hence the above design has been selected for illustration bearing in mind the fact that 20 comparisons between A and B are available, and that some of these may show no preference either way.

Once the design has been decided upon, the procedure in actual practice is to enter the results as they become available. In our example, the first patient, after his first and second doses, would have shown a preference for B. This is entered in the diagram by means of a line 1 unit in length (on the horizontal axis) moving downwards at 45°. The second patient had equal relief scores for A and B and would not therefore have entered the diagram. The third, fourth and fifth patients all showed preferences for B and would have been entered as

---

* This type of test, in which the possibility exists of a significant difference occurring in favour of either of the two drugs, is an example of the 'two-tailed test' referred to in the introduction to this Appendix.

further lines proceeding downwards at 45°. This would have been followed by a preference for *A*, and the graph would have been completed as in the illustration above.

It can be seen that a statistically significant difference in favour of *B* would have been demonstrated after 15 preferences and 4 ties, i.e. 19 patients altogether. In this example, therefore, there would have been no particular advantage in using a sequential method, since the study would have been terminated after 19 patients had been studied as opposed to 20 for the conventional methods of analysis.

First principles

Having looked at a number of statistical tests in a highly empirical manner, it may be interesting to return to a consideration of the probabilities involved in a study of this kind, arguing from first principles.

The point has been made in relation to the Chi-squared test that whereas the normal distribution and those distributions related to it are *continuous* distributions, the types of data that arise from analgesic trials are usually discontinuous. In our illustration, a patient's degree of relief may be represented as 2 or as 3, but it cannot be anything in between. The type of analysis appropriate for discontinuous data of this kind is based on the binomial distribution.

In our trial, every patient was given *A* and *B*. For each patient, various combinations of relief scores were possible: there may have been relief of 1 from *A* and 3 from *B*, 2 from *A* and 1 from *B* etc., etc. Altogether, there are 16 possibilities in each case, with the scoring system that was used, as is shown in Table A.8.

Of these 16 possible results, *A* is better than *B* in 6 cases, the relief scores are equal in 4 cases and *B* is better than *A* in 6 cases. The cases

Table A.8. Possible combinations of relief scores—score for *A* shown first

0	0	2	0
0	1*	2	1
0	2*	2	2
0	3*	2	3*
1	0	3	0
1	1	3	1
1	2*	3	2
1	3*	3	3

in which *B* is better than *A* are marked for convenience with asterisks in the above table.

If we adopt the 'null hypothesis' that *A* and *B* are not different, then it follows that all the 16 possible combinations of scores are equally probable in any one case. Therefore, if the 'null hypothesis' were true, the probability of *B* giving a better relief score than *A* in any one case would be $6 \div 16 = 0.375$.

What we actually observed was that in 20 cases, *B* gave a better relief score than *A* 15 times. What we clearly need to be able to do is to compare this observed finding with the probability that we would expect on the 'null hypothesis'.

Assuming the 'null hypothesis', the probability of *B* giving a better relief score than *A* 15 times out of 20 would be given by the 15th term of the binomial expansion $(p + q)^n$, where *p* is the probability of *B* proving better than *A* in a single case (0.375), *q* is the probability of *B* not proving better than *A* in a single case (i.e. $1 - p = 0.625$) and *n* is the number of cases studied.

In our example, the 15th term of the expansion would be

$$\frac{20!}{5! \times 15!} \times (0.375)^{15} \times (0.625)^5 = 0.000603$$

In the circumstances, this would clearly be a very unlikely event. We need to take account, however, not only of the *exact* probability of *B* coming out better 15 times, but also the probabilities of any *less likely* events (i.e. *B* proving better 16 or more times out of 20).

The full range of probabilities for the expansion

$$(0.375 + 0.625)^{20}$$

is shown in Table A.9.

From the Table A.9 it can be seen that the total probability of finding *B* to be better than *A* 15 times *or more* $= 0.000732$. This is therefore the probability of an event occurring in this particular 'tail' of the distribution. To make a 'two-tailed' estimate it would be necessary to take into account equally probable events in the other 'tail' of the distribution. In our case, inspection of the table shows that there is only one such event, namely the eventuality of *A* proving better than *B* in all 20 cases. Thus, the *total* probability of finding *B* better than *A* 15 times *or any less likely event* $= 0.000815$. All this, of course, relates to what the probabilities would be if *A* and *B* were in reality equally effective (the 'null hypothesis'). The probability that we have

Table A.9.

Number of times out of 20 that *B* is better than *A*	Probability
0	0·000083
1	0·000993
2	0·005658
3	0·020368
4	0·051939
5	0·099724
6	0·149586
7	0·179503
8	0·175016
9	0·140013
10	0·092408
11	0·050404
12	0·022682
13	0·008375
14	0·002512
15	0·000603
16	0·000113
17	0·000016
18	0·000000
19	0·000000
20	0·000000
Total	0·999996

arrived at is about once in one thousand two-hundred and thirty cases (i.e. $P < 0.001$), and we would be more than adequately justified in regarding this as a sufficiently unlikely event to reject the 'null hypothesis'.

The actual distribution of the probabilities listed in the above table can be represented graphically (Fig. A.3). This is a histogram of the expansion $(0.375 + 0.625)^{20}$. It illustrates an interesting and important point, namely that even when the probabilities p and q are unequal, the binomial distribution becomes symmetrical when n is sufficiently large. The above 'curve' approximates quite closely to a normal distribution.

The mean for a binomial distribution is given by

$$np = 20 \times 0.375$$

$$= 7.50$$

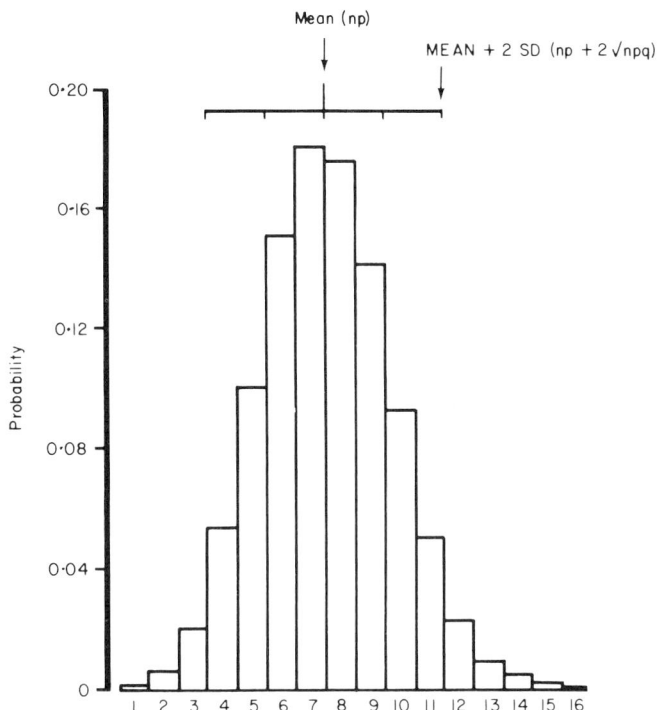

Fig. A.3. Distribution of probabilities: histogram of the expansion $(0.375 + 0.625)^{20}$.

Unlike the normal distribution, the binomial distribution has a standard deviation which is directly related to the mean,

$$SD = \sqrt{(npq)}$$
$$= 2.165$$

The mean plus and minus twice the standard deviation are shown on the above graph, and it can be seen that the value of 15 (i.e. the number of *B* preferences actually found) lies beyond 3 standard deviations from the mean.

In order to avoid the laborious computation of binomial probabilities, tables are available to which the observed results can be referred. Examples of such tables, with full textual explanation, are given by Mainland (1964).

Appendix 2

Opiates

a.i. Potent pure agonists

Drug	Trade name	Route	Dose 70 kg^{-1}	Duration
Morphine		s.c., i.m.	10 mg	4–5 h
		i.v.	4–10 mg	
		oral	8–20 mg	
Dextromoramide	Palfium	s.c., i.m.	5–10 mg	4–5 h
		oral	5–10 mg	
Dipipanone		s.c., i.m.	20–25 mg	4–5 h
	Diconal (+cyclizine HCl)	oral	10 mg	
Fentanyl	Sublimaze	i.v.	0·1–0·6 mg	2 h
Heroin		s.c., i.m.	5–10 mg	3–4 h
		oral	5–10 mg	
Levorphanol	Dromoran	s.c., i.m.	2–4 mg	4–5 h
		i.v.	1–1·5 mg	
		oral	1·5–4·5 mg	
Methadone	Physeptone	s.c., oral	5–10 mg	3–5 h
Oxycodone	Proladone	s.c.	5 mg	4–5 h
		oral	5–20 mg	
Pethidine		s.c., i.m.	25–100 mg	2–4 h
		i.v.	25–50 mg	
		oral	50–100 mg	
Phenazocine	Narphen	s.c., i.m.	1–3 mg	4–5 h
		i.v.	0·5–1 mg	
		oral	5–10 mg	
Phenoperidine	Operidine	i.v.	0·5–5 mg	1 h
Piritramide	Dipidolar	i.m.	20 mg	6 h

a.ii. Mild pure agonists

Drug	Trade name	Route	Dose 70 kg^{-1}	Duration
Codeine		oral	10–60 mg	4–6 h
Dihydrocodeine	DF 118	s.c., i.m.	30–60 mg	4–5 h
		oral	30–60 mg	
Ethoheptazine		oral	75–150 mg	4–6 h
Pholcodine		oral	Up to 60 mg	
d-Propoxyphene	Doloxene etc.	oral	65 mg	Up to 4 h

b. Narcotic antagonist analgesics

Drug	Trade name	Route	Dose 70 kg^{-1}	Duration
Buprenorphine	Temgesic	i.m.	0·3–0·6 mg	6–8 h
		slow i.v.	0·3–0·6 mg	6–8 h
Pentazocine	Fortral	s.c., i.m.	20–60 mg	3–4 h
		oral	25–100 mg	

c. Narcotic antagonists

Drug	Trade name	Route	Dose 70 kg^{-1}	Duration
Levallorphan	Lorphan	i.v.	0·5–1 mg	1–4 h
Nalorphine	Lethidrone	i.v.	5–10 mg	1–4 h
Naloxone	Narcan	i.v., i.m.	0·4–0·8 mg	0·75–1·5 h

d. Opiates with selectivity of action

Drug	Trade name	Route	Dose 70 kg^{-1}	Duration
Apomorphine (emetic)		s.c., i.m.	2–8 mg	
Dextromethorphan (antitussive)	Cosylan etc.	oral	15–30 mg	4–6 h
Diphenoxylate (constipative)	Lomotil	oral	2·5–10 mg	4–6 h

Appendix 2

Antipyretic analgesics

Drug	Trade name	Route	Dose 70 kg^{-1}	Duration:
Aspirin		oral	0·3–1 g	4–6 h
Diflunisal	Dolobid	oral	0·25–0·5 g	8–12 h
Mefenamic acid	Ponstan	oral	0·25–0·5 g	4–6 h
Flufenamic acid	Arlef	oral	0·1–0·3 g	4–6 h
Paracetamol	Panadol etc.	oral	0·5–1 g	4–6 h
Phenacetin		oral	0·3–0·6 g	4–6 h
Salicylamide	Salimed etc.	oral	0·3–1 g	4–8 h
Salicylic acid		oral	0·3–0·6 g	2–3 h

References

ABEL J.A. (1971) Analgesic nephropathy—A review of the literature, 1967–1970. *Clinical Pharmacology and Therapeutics*, **12**, 583–596.

ADAMS S.S. (1960) Analgesics—Antipyretics. *Journal of Pharmacy and Pharmacology*, **12**, 251–2.

AKIL H., MADDEN J., PATRICK R.L. & BARCHAS J.D. (1976) Stress induced increase in endogenous opiate peptides: Concurrent analgesia and its partial reversal by naloxone. In KOSTERLITZ H.W. (ed.) *Opiates and Endogenous Opioid Peptides.* Amsterdam, Elsevier/North Holland Biomedical Press, 63–70.

AKIL H., MAYER D.J. & LIEBESKIND J.C. (1976) Antagonism of stimulation-produced analgesia by naloxone, a narcotic antagonist. *Science*, **191**, 961–2.

ARMITAGE P. (1960) *Sequential Medical Trials.* Oxford, Blackwell Scientific Publications.

AXELROD J. (1956a) Possible mechanism of tolerance to narcotic drugs. *Science*, **124**, 263–4.

AXELROD J. (1956b) The enzymatic N-demethylation of narcotic drugs. *Journal of Pharmacology and Experimental Therapeutics*, **117**, 322–330.

BARNARDO D.E., CURREY H.L.F., MASON R.M., FOX W.R. & WEATHERALL M. (1966) Mefenamic Acid and Flufenamic Acid compared with Aspirin and Phenylbutazone in Rheumatoid Arthritis. *British Medical Journal*, **ii**, 342–3.

BAROWSKY H. & SCHWATZ S.A. (1962) Method for evaluating diphenoxylate hydrochloride. Comparison of its antidiarrheal effect with that of camphorated tincture of opium. *Journal of the American Medical Association*, **180**, 1058.

BATTERMAN R.C. (1963) Two point spacial discrimination device. *Proceedings of the Western Pharmacology Society*, **6**, 43–7.

BATTERMAN R.C. (1965) Persistence of responsiveness with placebo therapy following an effective drug trial. Paper presented at the *2nd Annual Meeting of The American College of Clinical Pharmacology and Chemotherapy, Chicago, Illinois, 3rd November.*

BEAVER W.T. (1965) Mild analgesics; A review of their clinical pharmacology. (Part I) *American Journal of Medical Science*, **250**, 577–604.

BEAVER W.T. (1966) Mild analgesics; A review of their clinical pharmacology. (Part II). *American Journal of Medical Science*, **251**, 576–599.

BEAVER W.T., WALLENSTEIN S.L., HOUDE R.W. & ROGERS A. (1968) A clinical comparison of the effects of oral and intramuscular administration of analgesics: Pentazocine and phenazocine. *Clinical Pharmacology and Therapeutics*, **9**, 582–597.

137

BECKETT A.H. & CASY A.F. (1954) Synthetic analgesics: Stereochemical considerations. *Journal of Pharmacy and Pharmacology*, **6**, 986–1001.

BECKETT A.H., CASY A.F. & HARPER N.J. (1956) Analgesics and their antagonists; some steric and chemical considerations. Part III. The influence of the basic group on the biological response. *Journal of Pharmacy and Pharmacology*, **8**, 874–884.

BECKETT A.H., TAYLOR J.F., CASY A.F. & HASSAN M.M.A. (1968) The biotransformation of methadone in man; synthesis and identification of a major metabolite. *Journal of Pharmacy and Pharmacology*, **20**, 754–762.

BEECHER H.K. (1955) The powerful placebo. *Journal of the American Medical Association*, **159**, 1602–6.

BEECHER H.K. (1957) The measurement of pain. Prototype for the quantitative study of subjective responses. *Pharmacological Reviews*, **9**, 59–209.

BEECHER H.K. & LASAGNA L. (1955) The analgesic effectiveness of nalorphine and nalorphine–morphine mixtures in man. *Journal of Pharmacology and Experimental Therapeutics*, **113**, 4–5.

BELL E.F. (1975) The use of naloxone in the treatment of diazepam poisoning. *Journal of Pediatrics*, **87**, 803–4.

BELLVILLE J.W., FORREST W.H. & BROWN B.W. (1968a) Clinical and statistical methodology for cooperative clinical assays of analgesics. *Clinical Pharmacology and Therapeutics*, **9**, 290–302.

BELLVILLE J.W., FORREST W.H., ELASHOFF J. & LASKA E. (1968b) Evaluating side effects of analgesics in a cooperative clinical study. *Clinical Pharmacology and Therapeutics*, **9**, 303–313.

BENNETT A., STAMFORD I.F. & UNGAR W.G. (1973) Prostaglandin E_2 and gastric acid secretion in man. *Journal of Physiology* (*London*), **229**, 349–360.

BENSON W.M., STEFKO P.L. & RANDALL L.O. (1953) Comparative pharmacology of levorphan, racemorphan and dextrorphan and related methyl esters. *Journal of Pharmacology and Experimental Therapeutics*, **109**, 189–200.

BERKOWITZ B.A. (1971) Influence of plasma levels and metabolism on pharmacological activity: Pentazocine. *Annals of the New York Academy of Science*, **179**, 269–281.

BERKOWITZ B.A., ASLING J.H., SHNIDER S.M. & WAY E.L. (1969) Relationship of pentazocine plasma levels to pharmacological activity in man. *Clinical Pharmacology and Therapeutics*, **10**, 320–8.

BERKOWITZ B.A., FINCK A.D. & NGAI S.H. (1977) Nitrous oxide analgesia: Reversal by naloxone and development of tolerance. *Journal of Pharmacology and Experimental Therapeutics*, **203**, 539–547.

BLACK W.P. (1966) Dangers of dextromoramide in obstetrical analgesia. *Practitioner*, **197**, 348–353.

BLATCHLY P.H. (1973) Naloxone for diagnosis in methadone programs. *Journal of the American Medical Association*, **224**, 334–5.

BLOOMQUIST E.R. (1963) The addiction potential of oxycodone (Percodan). *California Medicine*, **99**, 127–130.

BONEAU C.A. (1960) The effects of violations of assumptions underlying the test. *Psychological Bulletin*, **57**, 49–64.

BONICA J.J. (1953) *The Management of Pain*. London, Henry Kimpton, 115–128.

BONICA J.J. (1974) *Advances in Neurology. Volume 4: International Symposium on Pain.* New York, Raven Press.

BONICA J.J. & ALBE-FESSARD D. (1977) *Advances in Pain Research and Therapy. Volume 1,* New York, Raven Press.

BOROVSKY M.P. (1960) Antipyretic activity of acetylsalicylic acid and salicylamide suspension in pediatrics. A comparative clinical evaluation in two hundred and six cases. *American Medical Association Journal of Diseases of Children,* **100,** 23–30.

BOWSHER, D. (1977) The Anatomo-physiology of Pain. In LIPTON S. (ed.) *Persistent Pain: Modern Methods of Treatment.* Volume 1. London, Academic Press.

BOYD E.M. & BERECZKY G.M. (1966) Liver necrosis from paracetamol. *British Journal of Pharmacology,* **26,** 606–614.

BOYLE P. & PARBROOK G.D. (1977) The interrelation of personality and post operative factors. *British Journal of Anaesthesia,* **49,** 259–264.

BRADBURY A.F., SMYTH D.G., SNELL C.R., BIRDSALL N.J.M. & HULME E.C. (1976) C-fragment of lipotropin has a high affinity for brain opiate receptors. *Nature,* **260,** 793–5.

BRADLEY P.B., GAYTON R.J. & LAMBERT L.A. (1977) A microiontophoretic study of enkephalin and enkephalin analogues on brain stem neurones in the rat. *British Journal of Pharmacology,* **61,** 147–8P.

BRAHAM J., SAROVA-PINKAS I. & GOLDHAMMER Y. (1970) Apomorphine in parkinsonian tremor. *British Medical Journal,* iii, 768.

BRITTAIN G.J.C. (1959) Dihydrohydroxy-codeinone pectinate. *Lancet,* **2,** 544–6.

BRODIE B.B. & AXELROD J. (1948a) Estimation of acetanilide and its metabolic products, aniline, N-acetyl-p-aminophenol and p-aminophenol (free and total conjugated) in biological fluids and tissues. *Journal of Pharmacology and Experimental Therapeutics,* **94,** 22–8.

BRODIE B.B. & AXELROD J. (1948b) Fate of acetanilide in man. *Journal of Pharmacology and Experimental Therapeutics,* **94,** 29–38.

BRODIE B.B. & AXELROD J. (1949) The fate of acetophenetidin (phenacetin) in man and methods for the estimation of acetophenetidin and its metabolites in biological material. *Journal of Pharmacology and Experimental Therapeutics,* **97,** 58–67.

BROGDEN R.N., SPEIGHT T.M. & AVERY G.S. (1973) Pentazocine: A review of its pharmacological properties, therapeutic efficacy and dependence liability. *Drugs,* **5,** 6–91.

BROMAGE P.R. (1955) Spirometry in assessment of analgesia after abdominal surgery. A method of comparing analgesic drugs. *British Medical Journal,* ii, 589–593.

BROSS I.D.J. (1958) How to use RIDIT analysis. *Biometrics,* **14,** 18–38.

BROWN E.B. (1971) Drugs and respiratory control. *Annual Review of Pharmacology,* **11,** 271–284.

BUCHSBAUM M.S., DAVIS G.C. & BUNNEY W.E. (1977) Naloxone alters pain perception and somatosensory evoked potentials in normal subjects. *Nature,* **270,** 620–2.

CALDWELL J., WAKILE L.A., NOTARIANNI L.J., SMITH R.L., LIEBERMAN B.A., JEFFS J., COY Y. & BEARD R.W. (1977) Transplacental passage and neonatal elimination of pethidine given to mothers in childbirth. *British Journal of Clinical Pharmacology*, **4**, 715–6P.

CAMBELL C., PHILLIPS O.C. & FRAZIER T.M. (1961) Analgesia during labour: A comparison of pentobarbital, meperidine and morphine. *Obstetrics and Gynecology*, **17**, 714–8.

CASS L.J., FREDERIK W.S. & BARTHOLOMAY A.F. (1958) Methods of evaluating ethoheptazine combined with aspirin. *Journal of the American Medical Association*, **166**, 1829–1833.

CHAFEE F.H. & SETTIPANE G.A. (1974) Aspirin intolerance. I. Frequency in an allergic population. *Journal of Allergy and Clinical Immunology*, **53**, 193–9.

CHAPMAN C.R. (1974) An alternative to threshold assessment in the study of human pain. In BONICA J.J. (ed.) *Advances in Neurology. Volume 4: International Symposium on Pain.* New York, Raven Press, 115–121.

CLARK C.J. & DOWNIE C.C. (1966) A method for the rapid determination of the number of patients to include in a controlled clinical trial. *Lancet*, **ii**, 1357–8.

CLARK R.B., BEARD A.G. and BARCLAY D.L. (1975) Naloxone in the Newborn Infant. *Anesthesiology Review*, **2**, 9–11.

CLARK W.C. (1974) Pain sensitivity and the report of pain: an introduction to Sensory Decision Theory. *Anesthesiology*, **40**, 272–287.

CLARKE R.S.J. & DUNDEE J.W. (1965) Studies of drugs given before anaesthesia. IX Morphine with tacrine. *British Journal of Anaesthesia*, **37**, 779–784.

CLOUET D.H. (1971) Narcotic Drugs: Biochemical Pharmacology. New York, Plenum Press.

CLOUET D. & RATNER M. (1976) The incorporation of H^3-glycine into enkephalins in the brains of morphine treated rats. In KOSTERLITZ H.W. (ed.) *Opiates and Endogenous Opioid Peptides.* Amsterdam: Elsevier/North Holland Biomedical Press, 71–78.

CLUTTON-BROCK J. (1964) An improved device for measurement of the pain threshold. *Anaesthesia*, **19**, 593–5.

COHEN H. & JONES H.W. (1943) Reference of cardiac pain to a phantom left arm. *British Heart Journal*, **5**, 67–71.

COLGAN M.T. & MINTZ A.A. (1957) The comparative antipyretic effect of N-acetyl-p-aminophenol and acetylsalicylic acid. *Journal of Pediatrics*, **50**, 552–5.

COLLIER H.O.J. (1964) *Analgesics.* In LAURENCE D.R. & BACHARACH A.L. (eds.) *Evaluation of Drug Activities, Pharmacometrics.* Academic Press, New York, 183–203.

COLLIER H.O.J. (1969) A pharmacological analysis of aspirin. *Advances in Pharmacology and Chemotherapy*, **7**, 333–405.

COLLIER H.O.J. & SCHNEIDER C. (1972) Nociceptive responses to prostaglandins and analgesic actions of aspirin and morphine. *Nature New Biology*, **236**, 141–3.

CONNEY A.H., SANSUR M., SOROKO F., KOSTER R. & BURNS J.J. (1966) Enzyme induction and inhibition in studies on the pharmacological actions of acetophenetidin. *Journal of Pharmacology and Experimental Therapeutics*, **151**, 133–8.

COVE-SMITH J.R. & KNAPP M.S. (1978) Analgesic nephropathy: An important cause of chronic renal failure. *Quarterly Journal of Medicine. New Series*, **47**, 49–69.

COX B.M., GINSBURG M. & OSMAN O.H. (1968) Acute tolerance to narcotic analgesic drugs in rats. *British Journal of Pharmacology*, **33**, 245–256.

Cox B.M. & Weinstock M. (1966) The effect of analgesic drugs on the release of acetylcholine from electrically stimulated guinea pig ileum. *British Journal of Pharmacology*, **27**, 81–92.

Cranston W.I., Hellon R.F., Luff R.H., Rawlins M.D. & Rosendorff C. (1970) Observations on the mechanism of salicylate induced antipyresis. *Journal of Physiology (London)*, **210**, 593–600.

Cummings A.J. & Martin B.K. (1968) Interpretation of the kinetics of salicylic acid elimination. *Journal of Pharmaceutical Sciences*, **57**, 891–3.

D'Amour F.E. & Smith D.L. (1941) A method for determining loss of pain sensation. *Journal of Pharmacology and Experimental Therapeutics*, **72**, 74–9.

Davey E.A. and Murray J.B. (1969) Hydrolysis of diamorphine in aqueous solutions. *Pharmaceutical Journal*, **203**, 737.

David M. & Deligné P. (1957) Un nouvel analgésique de synthèse: Le R 875. *La Presse Médicale*, **65**, 731–3.

Davidson D.G.D. & Eastham W.N. (1966) Acute liver necrosis following overdose of paracetamol. *British Medical Journal*, **ii**, 497–9.

Deneau G.A. & Nakai K. (1961) The toxicity of meperidine in the monkey as influenced by its rate of absorption. In *Minutes of the 23rd Meeting of the Committee on Drug Addiction and Narcotics. Appendix 6 NAS-NRC*, Washington, D.C.

Dettmar P.W., Cowan A. & Walter D.S. (1978) Naloxone antagonises behavioural effects of d-amphetamine in mice and rats. *Neuropharmacology*, **17**, 1041–1044.

Dixon M.F. (1976) Paracetamol hepatotoxicity. *Lancet*, **i**, 35.

Dole V.P. & Kreek M.J. (1973) Methadone plasma levels sustained by a reservoir of drug in tissue. *Proceedings of the National Academy of Sciences of the United States of America*, **70**, 10.

Done A.K. (1959) Uses and abuses of antipyretic therapy. *Pediatrics (Springfield)*, **23**, 774–780..

Done A.K. (1969) Pharmacological principles in the treatment of poisoning. *Pharmacology for Physicians*, **3**, 1–10.

Douglas A.P., Hamlyn A.N. & James O. (1976) Controlled trial of cysteamine in treatment of acute paracetamol (acetaminophen) poisoning. *Lancet*, **i**, 111–5.

Downes J.J., Kemp R.A. & Lambertsen C.J. (1967) The magnitude and duration of respiratory depression due to fentanyl and meperidine in man. *Journal of Pharmacology and Experimental Therapeutics*, **158**, 416–420.

Dripps R.D. & Comroe J.H. (1945) Clinical studies of morphine. I. The immediate effect of morphine administered intravenously and intramuscularly upon the respiration of normal man. *Anesthesiology*, **6**, 462–8.

Dubas T.C. & Parker J.M. (1971) A central component in the analgesic action of sodium salicylate. *Archives internationales de Pharmacodynamie et de Therapie*, **194**, 117–122.

Dunbar B.S., Ovassapian A., Dripps R.D. & Smith T.C. (1967) The respiratory response to carbon dioxide during INNOVAR-nitrous oxide anaesthesia in man. *British Journal of Anaesthesia*, **39**, 861–6.

Duncan D.B. (1955) Multiple range and multiple F tests. *Biometrics*, **11**, 1–42.

DUNDEE J.W. (1960) Alteration in response to somatic pain associated with anaesthesia. II The effect of thiopentone and pentobarbitone. *British Journal of Anaesthesia*, **32**, 407–414.

DYRBERG V., HENNINGSEN P. & JOHANSEN S.H. (1967) The respiratory effects of pentazocine. *Acta Anaesthesiologica Scandinavica*, **11**, 77–84.

ECONOMOU G., MONSON R. & WARD-McQUAID J.N. (1971) Oral pentazocine and phenazocine: A comparison in post operative pain. *British Journal of Anaesthesia*, **43**, 486–495.

EDDY N.B. (1932) Studies of morphine, codeine and their derivatives. I: General methods. *Journal of Pharmacology and Experimental Therapeutics*, **45**, 339–359.

EDDY N.B., FRIEBEL H., HAHN K-J. & HALBACH H. (1970) Codeine and its alternatives for pain and cough relief. Genève, World Health Organization.

EGBERT L.D., BATTIT G.E., WELCH C.E. & BARTLETT M.K. (1964) Reduction of postoperative pain by encouragement and instruction of patients. *New England Journal of Medicine*, **270**, 825–7.

ERNST A.M. (1967) Mode of action of apomorphine and dexamphetamine on gnawing compulsion in rats. *Psychopharmacologia*, **10**, 316–323.

EVANS L.E.J., SWAINSON C.P., ROSCOE P. & PRESCOTT L.F. (1973) Treatment of drug overdosage with naloxone, a specific narcotic antagonist. *Lancet*, **i**, 452–455.

EVANS J.M., HOGG M.I.J., LUNN J.N. & ROSEN M. (1974) A comparative study of the narcotic agonist activity of naloxone and levallorphan. *Anaesthesia*, **29**, 721–7.

EVANS W.O. (1962) A comparison of the analgesic potency of some analgesics as measured by the 'Flinch-Jump' procedure. *Psychopharmacologia*, **3**, 51–54.

FELDBERG W. & MILTON A.S. (1973) Postaglandin Fever. In SCHONBAUM E. & LOMAX P. (eds) *The Pharmacology of Thermoregulation. Basel, Karger*, 302–310.

FERREIRA S.H., MONCADA S. & VANE J.R. (1971) Indomethacin and aspirin abolishes prostaglandin release from the spleen. *Nature*, **231**, 237–9.

FERREIRA S.H. & VANE J.R. (1974) New aspects of the mode of action of nonsteroid anti-inflammatory drugs. *Annual Review of Pharmacology*, **14**, 57–73.

FERTSIGER A.P. & FISCHER R. (1977) Interaction between narcotic antagonist (naloxone) and lysergic acid diethylamine in the rat. *Psychopharmacology*, **54**, 313–4.

FINCH J.S. & DeKORNFELD T.J. (1967) Clinical investigation of the analgesic potency and respiratory depressant activity of fentanyl: A new narcotic analgesic. *Journal of Clinical Pharmacology*, **7**, 46–51.

FLACKE J.W., FLACKE W.E. & WILLIAMS G.D. (1977) Acute pulmonary edema following naloxone reversal of high dose morphine anesthesia. *Anesthesiology*, **47**, 376–8.

FLOREZ J. & MEDIAVILLA A. (1977) Respiratory and cardiovascular effects of met-enkephalin applied to the ventral surface of the brain stem. *Brain Research*, **138**, 585–590.

FLOREZ J., McCARTHY L.E. & BORISON H.L. (1968) A comparative study in the cat of the respiratory effects of morphine injected intravenously and into the cerebrospinal fluid. *Journal of Pharmacology and Experimental Therapeutics*, **163**, 448–455.

FLOWER R.J. & VANE J.R. (1972) Inhibitors of prostaglandin synthetase in brain explains the antipyretic activity of paracetamol (4-Acetamidophenol). *Nature*, **240**, 410–411.

FLOWER R.J., GRYGLEWSKI R., HERBACZYŃSKA-CEDRO K. & VANE J.R. (1972) Effects of anti-inflammatory drugs on prostaglandin biosynthesis. *Nature New Biology,* **238**, 104–6.

FOLDES F.F. (1973) Use of narcotic antagonists during labour and delivery. In *Bases fondamentales de l'Anaesthésie et de la Réanimation Obstétricales. Société francais d'Anesthésie, d'Analgésie et de Réanimation,* 4. Paris, Librairie Arnett, 370–377.

FOLDES F.F., KEPES E.R., TORDA T.A.G., BAILEY R. & WULFSOHN N.L. (1964) Clinico-pharmacological studies with fentanyl and droperidol. In *Proceedings of the 3rd World Congress of Anaesthesiology (Sao Paulo),* **2**, 239.

FOLDES F.F., SWERDLOW M. & SIKER E.S. (1964) *Narcotics and narcotic antagonists Chemistry, pharmacology and applications in anaesthesiology and obstetrics.* 1st edition 192. Illinois, Thomas.

FOLDES F.F. & TORDA T.A.G. (1965) Comparative studies with narcotic antagonists in man. *Acta Anaesthesiologica Scandinavica,* **9**, 121–138.

FORREST W.H., BEER E.G., BELVILLE J.W., CILIBERTI B.J., MILLER E.V. & PADDOCK R. (1969) Analgesic and other effects of the d- and l-isomers of pentazocine. *Clinical Pharmacology and Therapeutics,* **10**, 468–476.

FOX J.W.C., FOX E.J. & CRANDELL D.L. (1967) Neuroleptanalgesia for heart and major surgery. *Archives of Surgery,* **94**, 102–6.

FREDERICKSON R.C.A. (1977) Enkephalin pentapeptides—A review of current evidence for a physiological role in vertebrate neurotransmission. *Life Sciences,* **21**, 23–42.

FREY G.H. (1961) The role of placebo responses in clinical headache evaluation. *Headache,* **1**, 31–8.

FREY M. VON (1895) Beitrage zur sinnesphysiologie der haut. *Dritte Mittheilung Berichte uber die Verhandlungen der Koniglich Sachsischen Gesellschaft der Wissenschaffen zu Leipzig. Mathematisch-Physische Classe,* **47**, 166–184.

FRASER H.F. & ISBELL H. (1961) Human pharmacology and addictiveness of ethyl 1-(3-cyano-3,3-phenylpropyl)-4-phenyl-4-piperide carboxylate hydrochloride (R-1132 diphenoxylate). *Bulletin on Narcotics (New York),* **13**, 29–43.

GLASER F.B. & BALL J.C. (1970) Death due to withdrawal from narcotics. In BALL J.C. & CHAMBERS C.D. (eds.) *The Epidemiology of Opiate Addiction in the United States.* Springfield, Charles C. Thomas, 263–287.

GOODMAN L.S. & GILMAN A. (1975) *The Pharmacological Basis of Therapeutics.* 5th Edition. New York, Macmillan Publishing Co., Inc.

GRAFFENRIED B. VON, POZO E. DEL., ROUBICEK J., KREBS E., POLDINGER W., BUR-MEISTER P. & KERP L. (1978) Effects of the synthetic enkephalin analogue FK 33–824 in man. *Nature,* **272**, 729–730.

GUNNE L-M., LINDSTROM L. & TERENIUS L. (1977) Naloxone induced reversal of schizophrenia hallucinations. *Journal of Neural Transmission,* **40**, 13–9.

GUTNER L.B., GOULD W.J. & BATTERMAN R.C. (1952) The effects of potent anal-gesics upon vestibular function. *Journal of Clinical Investigation,* **31**, 259–266.

GWILT J.R., ROBERTSON A., GOLDMAN L. & BLANCHARD A.W. (1963) The absorption characteristics of paracetamol tablets in man. *Journal of Pharmacy and Pharma-cology,* **15**, 445–453.

GYÖRY A.Z. & STIEL J.N. (1968) Effect of particle size on aspirin induced gastro-intestinal bleeding. *Lancet,* **ii**, 300–2.

HAFFNER F. (1929) Experimentelle prufüng schmerzstellender mittel. *Deutsche Medizinische Wochenschrift*, **55**, 731–3.

HAJNAL J., SHARP J. & POPERT A.J. (1959) A method for testing analgesics in rheumatoid arthritis using a sequential procedure. *Annals of the Rheumatic Diseases (London)*, **18**, 189–206.

HARDY J.D., WOLFF H.G. & GOODELL H. (1940) Studies on pain. A new method for measuring pain threshold: Observations on spatial summation of pain. *Journal of Clinical Investigation*, **19**, 649–657.

HARVEY S.C. (1975) Hypnotics and sedatives. The barbiturates. In GOODMAN L.S. & GILMAN A. (eds) *The Pharmacological Basis of Therapeutics*. New York, Macmillan Publishing Co., Inc., 118.

HASSLER R. (1972) The division of pain conduction into systems of pain sensation and pain awareness. In PAYNE J.P. & BURT R.A.P. (eds.) *Pain: Basic Principles-Pharmacology-Therapy*. London, Churchill Livingstone, 98–112.

HEAD H. & HOLMES G. (1912a) Researches into sensory disturbances from cerebral lesions II. *Lancet*, **i**, 79–83.

HEAD H. & HOLMES G. (1912b) Researches into sensory disturbances from cerebral lesions III. *Lancet*, **i**, 144–152.

HENDERSON G., HUGHES J. & KOSTERLITZ H.W. (1972) A new example of a morphine sensitive neuroeffector junction: Adrenergic transmission in the mouse vas deferens. *British Journal of Pharmacology*, **46**, 764–6.

HERTZ A., ALBUS K., METYS J., SHUBERT P. & TESCHEMACHER H. (1970) On the central sites for the antinociceptive actions of morphine and fentanyl. *Neuropharmacology*, **9**, 539–551.

HILL J.B. (1973) Salicylate intoxication. *New England Journal of Medicine*, **288**, 1110–3.

HOGBEN C.A., SCHANKER L.S., TOCCO D.J. & BRODIE B.B. (1957) Absorption of drugs from the stomach. II. The human. *Journal of Pharmacology and Experimental Therapeutics*, **120**, 540–5.

HORN A.S. & RODGERS J.R. (1977) The enkephalin and opiate structure activity relations. *Journal of Pharmacy and Pharmacology*, **29**, 257–265.

HUGHES J. (1975) Isolation of an endogenous compound from the brain with pharmacological properties similar to morphine. *Brain Research*, **88**, 295–308.

HUGHES J., KOSTERLITZ H.W. & SMITH T.W. (1977) The distribution of methionine-enkephalin and leucine-enkephalin in the brain and peripheral tissues. *British Journal of Pharmacology*, **61**, 639–647.

HUGHES J., SMITH T.W., KOSTERLITZ H.W., FOTHERGILL L.A., MORGAN B.A. & MORRIS, H.R. (1975) Identification of two related pentapeptides from the brain with potent opiate agonist activity. *Nature*, **258**, 577–9.

HUNTER A.R., PLEUVRY B.J. & REES J.M.H. (1968) The respiratory depressant effects of barbituates and narcotic analgesics in the unanaesthetized rabbit. *British Journal of Anaesthesia*, **40**, 927–935.

HUTCHINSON M., KOSTERLITZ H. W., LESLIE F.M., WATERFIELD A.A. & TERENIUS L. (1975) Assessment in the guinea pig ileum and mouse vas deferens of benzomorphans which have strong antinociceptive activity but do not substitute for morphine in the dependent monkey. *British Journal of Pharmacology*, **55**, 541–6.

IGGO A. (1972) The case for 'pain' receptors. In PAYNE J.P. & BURT R.A.P. (eds.). *Pain: Basic Principles-Pharmacology-Therapy*. London, Churchill Livingstone, 60–7.

IGGO A. (1976) Peripheral and spinal 'pain' mechanisms and their modulation. In BONICA J.J. and ALBE-FESSARD D. (eds.) *Advances in Pain Research and Therapy*. New York, Raven Press, 381–394.

JACQUET Y.F. & LAJTHA A. (1973) Morphine action at central nervous sites in rat: Analgesia or hyperalgesia depending on site and dose. *Science*, **182**, 490–492.

JAFFE J.H. (1975) Drug addiction and drug abuse. In GOODMAN L.S. & GILMAN A. (eds.) *The Pharmacological Basis of Therapeutics*. New York. Macmillan Publishing Co. Inc., 284–324.

JAFFE J.H. & MARTIN W.R. (1975) Narcotic analgesics and antagonists. In GOODMAN L.S. & GILMAN A. (eds.) *The Pharmacological Basis of Therapeutics*, New York, Macmillan Publishing Co., Inc., 251, 258.

JAMES W. (1890) *The Principles of Psychology. Volume 1.* Reprinted 1950, Dover Publications Inc., 190.

JANSSEN P.A.J. (1968) Chemical structure and morphinomimetic activity. In SOULAIRAC A., CAHN J. & CHARPENTIER J. (eds.) *Pain*. New York, Academic Press, 233–238.

JELLINEK E.M. (1946) Clinical tests on comparative effectiveness of analgesic drugs. *Biometrics Bulletin*, **2**, 87–91.

JENNETT S., BARKER J.G. & FORREST J.B. (1968) A double blind controlled study of the effects on respiration of pentazocine, phenoperidine and morphine in normal man. *British Journal of Anaesthesia*, **40**, 864–875.

JESSELL T.M. & IVERSEN L.L. (1977) Opiate analgesics inhibit substance P release from rat trigeminal nucleus. *Nature*, **268**, 549–551.

JOHNSTONE C.M. (1958) Dipipanone hydrochloride (Pipadone) as a pre-delivery sedative and analgesic. *Canadian Medical Association Journal*, **79**, 488–9.

JOLLOW D.J., MITCHELL J.R., POTTER W.Z., DAVIS D.C., GILLETTE J.R. & BRODIE B.B. (1973) Acetaminophen-induced hepatic necrosis II. Role of covalent binding *in vivo*. *Journal of Pharmacology and Experimental Therapeutics*, **187**, 195–202.

KALLOS T. & SMITH T.C. (1969) The respiratory effects of innovar given for pre-medication. *British Journal of Anaesthesia*, **41**, 303–6.

KARIM A., RANNEY R.E., EVENSEN K.L. & CLARK M.L. (1972) Pharmacokinetics and metabolism of diphenoxylate in man. *Clinical Pharmacology and Therapeutics*, **13**, 407–419.

KEATS A.S. (1969) Discussion in a Research Symposium on the Evaluation of Strong Analgesics. *Clinical Trials Journal (Special Issue)*, **6**, 126.

KEATS A.S., BEECHER H.K. & MOSTELLER F.C. (1950) Measurement of pathological pain in distinction to experimental pain. *Journal of Applied Physiology*, **3**, 35–44.

KEATS A.S. & TELFORD J. (1964) Studies of analgesic drugs. VIII. A narcotic antagonist without psychotomimetic effects. *Journal of Pharmacology and Experimental Therapeutics*, **143**, 157–164.

KEATS A.S., TELFORD J. & KUROSU Y. (1957) Studies of analgesic drugs: Dihydrocodeine. *Journal of Pharmacology and Experimental Therapeutics*, **120**, 354–360.

KEELE C.A. & ARMSTRONG D. (1964) *Substances producing pain and itch*. London, Edward Arnold Ltd., 399.

KEELE K.D. (1948) The pain chart. *Lancet*, **ii**, 6–8.

KELLGREN J.H. (1969) Pain. In COPEMAN W.S.C. (ed.) *Textbook of Rheumatic Diseases* 4th edition. Edinburgh, E. & S. Livingstone Ltd. 18–39.

KERSH E.S. (1973) Treatment of propoxyphene overdosage with naloxone. *Chest*, **63**, 112–4.

KING A. & BETTS T.A. (1978) Abuse of pentazocine. *British Medical Journal*, **ii**, 21.

KOSTERLITZ H.W., COLLIER H.O.J. & VILLARREAL J.E. (1972) *Agonist and antagonist actions of narcotic analgesic drugs.* London, Macmillan.

KOSTERLITZ H.W., LORD J.A.H. & WATT A.J. (1973) Morphine receptors in the myenteric plexus of the guinea pig ileum. In KOSTERLITZ H.W., COLLIER H.O.J. & VILLARREAL J.E. (eds.) *Agonist and antagonist actions of narcotic analgesic drugs.* London, Macmillan, 45–61.

KOSTERLITZ H.W. & WATERFIELD A.A. (1975) *In vitro* models in the study of structure activity relationships of narcotic analgesics. *Annual Review of Pharmacology*, **15**, 29–47.

KOSTERLITZ H.W. & WATT A.J. (1968) Kinetic parameters of narcotic agonists and antagonists with particular reference to N-allyl-noroxymorphone (naloxone). *British Journal of Pharmacology*, **33**, 266–276.

KRAMER C.Y. (1956) Extension of multiple range tests to group means with unequal numbers of replications. *Biometrics*, **12**, 307–310.

KREUGER H., EDDY N.B. & SUMWALT M. (1941) *The pharmacology of the opium alkaloids Part 1* (U.S. Public Health Reports. Supplement 165) Washington, D.C., U.S. Government Printing Office.

KUHAR M.J., PERT C.B. & SNYDER S.H. (1973) Regional distribution of opiate receptor binding in monkey and human brain. *Nature*, **245**, 447–450.

LAMBERTSEN C.J. (1966) Drugs and respiration. *Annual Review of Pharmacology*, **6**, 327–378.

LASAGNA L. (1960) The clinical measurement of pain. *Annals of the New York Academy of Science*, **86**, 28–37.

LASAGNA L. (1964) The clinical value of morphine and its substitutes as analgesics. *Pharmacological Reviews*, **16**, 47–83.

LASAGNA L. & BEECHER H.K. (1954) The analgesic effectiveness of nalorphine and nalorphine-morphine combinations in man. *Journal of Pharmacology and Experimental Therapeutics*, **112**, 356–363.

LASAGNA L., DAVIS M. & PEARSON J.W. (1967) A comparison of acetophenetidin and acetaminophen. I Analgesic effects in post partum patients. *Journal of Pharmacology and Experimental Therapeutics*, **155**, 296–300.

LASAGNA L., VON FELSINGER J.M. & BEECHER H.K. (1955) Drug-induced mood changes in man. 1. Observations on healthy subjects, chronically ill patients and 'Postaddicts'. *Journal of the American Medical Association*, **157**, 1006–1020.

LASAGNA L., MOSTELLER F., VON FELSINGER J.M. & BEECHER H.K. (1954) A study of placebo response. *The American Journal of Medicine*, **16**, 770–9.

LELE P.P. & WEDDELL G. (1959) Sensory nerves of the cornea and cutaneous sensibility. *Experimental Neurology*, **1**, 334–359.

LEMBERGER L. & RUBIN A. (1976) Physiologic disposition of drugs of abuse, pp. 125–161. New York: Spectrum Publications.

LEONARDS J.R. & LEVY G. (1969) Reduction or prevention of aspirin induced occult gastrointestinal blood loss in man. *Clinical Pharmacology and Therapeutics*, **10**, 571–5.

LESNA M., WATSON A.J., DOUGLAS A.P.,HAMLYN A.N. & JAMES O. (1976) Toxicity of paracetamol. *Lancet*, **1**, 191.

LEVINE J.D., GORDON N.C., JONES R.T. & FIELDS H.L. (1978) The narcotic antagonist naloxone enhances clinical pain. *Nature*, **272**, 826–7.

LEVY M. (1974) Aspirin use in patients with major upper gastrointestinal bleeding and peptic ulcer disease. *New England Journal of Medicine*, **290**, 1158–1162.

LITTLE H.J. & REES J.M.H. (197) Naloxone antagonism of sympathomimetic analgesia. In VAN REE J.M. & TERENIUS L. (eds.) *Characteristics and function of opioids*. Amsterdam, Elsevier/North Holland Biomedical Press. 433–4.

LOH H.H., CHO T.M. WU Y-C. & WAY E.L. (1974) Stereospecific binding of narcotics to brain cerebrosides. *Life Sciences*, **14**, 2231–2245.

MAHER R.M. (1975) Cancer pain in relation to nursing care, *Nursing Times*, **71**, 344–350.

MAINLAND D. (1964) Composite Indices—What do they indicate? Notes from a Laboratory of Medical Statistics. *Notes*, 73–77.

MANDEL H.G., RODWELL V.W. & SMITH P.K. (1952) A study of the metabolism of C^{14} salicylamide in the human. *Journal of Pharmacology and Experimental Therapeutics*, **106**, 433–9.

MARTIN W.R. (1967) Opioid antagonists. *Pharmacological Reviews*, **19**, 463–521.

MARTIN W.R., EADES C.G., THOMPSON J.A., HUPPLER R.E. & GILBERT P.E. (1976) The effects of morphine and nalorphine like drugs in the nondependent and morphine dependent chronic spinal dog. *Journal of Pharmacology and Experimental Therapeutics*, **197**, 517–533.

MATTS S.G.F., SWAN C.H.J. & WHARTON B.A. (1964) Double blind trial of dextromoramide methadone and pethidine in the treatment of severe pain. *Postgraduate Medical Journal*, **40**, 103–5.

MAXWELL A.E. (1961) *Analysing qualitative data*. London, Methuen & Co. Ltd.

MAXWELL C. (1978) Sensitivity and accuracy of the visual analogue scale: a psychophysical classroom experiment. *British Journal of Clinical Pharmacology*, **6**, 15–24.

MAYER D.J. & PRICE D.D. (1976) Central nervous system mechanisms of analgesia. *Pain*, **2**, 374–404.

MELZAK R. & WALL P.D. (1965) Pain mechanisms: A new theory. *Science*, **150**, 971–979.

MICHAELIS L.L., HICKEY P.R., CLARK T.A. & DIXON W.M. (1974) Ventricular irritability associated with the use of naloxone hydrochloride. *The Annals of Thoracic Surgery*, **18**, 608–621.

MILLER R.R., FEINGOLD A. & PAXINOS J. (1970) Propoxyphene hydrochloride. A critical review. *Journal of the American Medical Association*, **213**, 996–1006.

MITCHELL J.R., JOLLOW D.J., POTTER W.Z., DAVIS D.C., GILLETTE J.R. & BRODIE B.B. (1973a) Acetaminophen induced hepatic necrosis. I. Role of drug metabolism. *Journal of Pharmacology and Experimental Therapeutics*, **187**, 185–194.

MITCHELL J.R., JOLLOW D.J., POTTER W.Z., GILLETTE J.R. & BRODIE B.B. (1973b) Acetaminophen induced hepatic necrosis. IV. Protective role of glutathione. *Journal of Pharmacology and Experimental Therapeutics*, **187**, 211–7.

MOERTAL C.G., AHMANN D.L., TAYLOR W.F. & SCHWATAU N. (1972) A comparative evaluation of marketed analgesic drugs. *New England Journal of Medicine*, **286**, 813–5.

MOERTAL C.G., AHMANN D.L., TAYLOR W.F. & SCHWARTAU N. (1974) Relief of pain by oral medications. A controlled evaluation of analgesic combinations. *Journal of the American Medical Association*, **229**, 55–9.

MOORE J. & DUNDEE J.W. (1961) Alteration in response to somatic pain associated with anaesthesia. V. The effect of promethazine. *British Journal of Anaesthesia*, **33**, 3–8.

MORGAN M., LUMLEY J. & GILLIES I.D.S. (1974) Neuroleptanaesthesia for major surgery: experience with 500 cases. *British Journal of Anaesthesia*, **46**, 288–293.

MORONEY M.J. (1951) Facts from Figures. Harmondsworth Middlesex, Penguin Books.

MORRISON J.D., LOAN W.B. & DUNDEE J.W. (1971) Controlled comparison of the efficacy of 14 preparations in the relief of post-operative pain. *British Medical Journal*, iii, 287–290.

MOSS L.M. (1973) Naloxone reversal of non-narcotic induced apnea. *Journal of the American College of Emergency Physicians*, **2**, 46–48.

MOYNIHAN N.H. (1965) The treatment of alcoholism in general practice. *Practitioner*, **195**, 223–7.

MULÉ S.J. (1971) Physiological disposition of narcotic agonists and antagonists. In CLOUET D.H. (ed.) *Narcotic Drugs, Biochemical Pharmacology*. New York, Plenum Press, 99–121.

MURRAY T. & GOLDBERG M. (1975) Analgesic abuse and renal disease. *Annual Review of Medicine*, **26**, 537–550.

MUSTARD J.F. & PACKMAN M.A. (1970) Factors influencing platelet function, adhesion, release and aggregation. *Pharmacological Reviews*, **22**, 97–187.

NAKAHAMA H. (1975) Pain mechanisms in the central nervous system. *International Anesthesiology Clinics*, **13**, 109–148.

NICHOLSON A.N. (1978) Visual analogue scales and drug effects in man. *British Journal of Clinical Pharmacology*, **6**, 3–4.

NOORDENBOS W. (1959) Pain: Problems pertaining to the transmission of nerve impulses which give rise to pain. Amsterdam, Elsevier Publishing Co.

ORKIN L.R., EGGE R.K. & ROVENSTINE E.A. (1955) Effect of Nisentil, meperidine and morphine on respiration in man. *Anesthesiology*, **16**, 699–707.

OVERHOLT R.H. (1930) Postoperative pulmonary hypoventilation. *Journal of the American Medical Association*, **95**, 1484–1489.

PAPPER E.M., BRODIE B.B. & ROVENSTINE E.A. (1952) Postoperative pain, its use in the comparative evaluation of analgesics. *Surgery*, **32**, 107–9.

PARKHOUSE J. (1963) Placebo Reactor. *Nature*, **199**, 308.

PARKHOUSE J. (1967) Recording and analysis of clinical data. *British Journal of Anaesthesia*, **39**, 35–7.

PARKHOUSE J. & HALLINON P. (1967) A comparison of aspirin and paracetamol. With a note on method. *British Journal of Anaesthesia*, **39**, 146–154.

PARKHOUSE J., HENRIE J.R., DUNCAN G.M. & ROME H.P. (1960) Nitrous oxide analgesia in relation to mental performance. *Journal of Pharmacology and Experimental Therapeutics*, **128**, 44–54.

PARKHOUSE J. & HOLMES C.M. (1963) Assessing post operative pain relief. *Proceedings of the Royal Society of Medicine*, **56**, 579–584.

PARKHOUSE J., LAMBRECHTS W. & SIMPSON B.R.J. (1961) The incidence of postoperative pain. *British Journal of Anaesthesia*, **33**, 345–353.

PARKHOUSE J. & WRIGHT V. (1968) Postoperative analgesia with CI-572. *Canadian Medical Association Journal*, **99**, 887–891.

PATTON H.D. (1974) Floor Discussion: Pain threshold. In BONICA J.J. (ed.) *Advances in Neurology. Volume 4: International Symposium on Pain.* New York, Raven Press. 123–6.

PAULUS H.E. & WHITEHOUSE M.W. (1973) Non steroid anti-inflammatory agents. *Annual Review of Pharmacology*, **13**, 107–125.

PAYNE J.P. & BURT R.A.P. (1972) *Pain: Basic Principles—Pharmacology—Therapy.* London, Churchill Livingstone.

PEÑA E. (1965) Comparison of oral promethazine-meperidine with injectable meperidine for relief of postoperative pain. *Obstetrics and Gynecology*, **25**, 72–5.

PENTIAH P., REILLY F. & BORISON H.L. (1966) Interactions of morphine sulphate and sodium salicylate on respiration in cats. *Journal of Pharmacology and Experimental Therapeutics*, **154**, 110–18.

PERT A. (1975) Analgesia produced by morphine microinjections in primate brain. In SNYDER S.H. & MATTHYSSE S. (eds.) *Opiate Receptor Mechanisms.* Cambridge (Mass.), MIT Press, 87–91.

PERT A. & YAKSH T. (1974) Sites of morphine induced analgesia in the primate brain: relation to pain pathways. *Brain Research*, **80**, 135–140.

PICKERING G.W. (1949) The place of the experimental method in medicine. *Proceeding of the Royal Society of Medicine*, **42**, 229–234.

POMERANZ B. (1977) Brain opiates at work in acupuncture. *New Scientist*, **73**, 12–3.

POMERANZ B. & CHIU D. (1976) Naloxone blockade of acupuncture analgesia: Endorphin implicated. *Life Science*, **19**, 1757–1762.

POTTER W.Z., DAVIS D.C., MITCHELL J.R., JOLLOW D.J., GILLETTE J.R. & BRODIE B.B. (1973) Acetaminophen induced hepatic necrosis. III Cytochrome P450 mediated covalent binding *in vivo. Journal of Pharmacology and Experimental Therapeutics*, **187**, 203–210.

PRESCOTT L.F. (1965) Effects of acetylsalicylic acid, phenacetin, paracetamol and caffeine on renal tubular epithelium. *Lancet*, **ii**, 91–6.

PRESCOTT L.F., HOWIE D., DARRIEN I. & ADRIAENSSENS P. (1977) Paracetamol hepatotoxicity in man. In *Alfred Benzon Symposium X: Drug design and adverse reactions.* Copenhagen, Munksgaard, 99–109.

PRESCOTT L.F., NEWTON R.W., SWAINSON C.P., WRIGHT N., FORREST A.R.W. & MATTHEW H. (1974) Successful treatment of severe paracetamol overdosage with cysteamine. *Lancet*, **i**, 588–592.

PRESCOTT L.F. & WRIGHT N. (1973) The effects of hepatic and renal damage on paracetamol metabolism and excretion following overdosage. A pharmacokinetic study. *British Journal of Pharmacology*, **49**, 602–613.

150 *References*

PROUDFOOT A.T. & WRIGHT N. (1970) Acute paracetamol poisoning. *British Medical Journal*, iii, 557–8.

PUIG M.M., GASCON P., CRAVISO G.L. & MUSACCHIO J.M. (1977) Endogenous opiate receptor ligand: Electrically induced release in the guinea pig ileum. *Science*, **195**, 419–420.

QUICK A.J. & CLESCERI L. (1960) Influence of acetylsalicylic acid and salicylamide on the coagulation of blood. *Journal of Pharmacology and Experimental Therapeutics*, **128**, 95–98.

RANDALL L.O. (1963) Non-narcotic analgesics. In ROOT W.S. & HOFMANN F.G. (eds.) *Physiological Pharmacology*, Volume 1. New York, Academic Press, 313–416.

RANDALL L.O. & SELITTO J.J. (1957) A method for measurement of analgesic activity on inflamed tissue. *Archives Internationales de Pharmacodynamie et de Thérapie*, **111**, 409–419.

RANDALL L.O. & SELITTO J.J. (1958) Anti-inflammatory effects of Romilar CF. *Journal of the American Pharmaceutical Association Scientific Edition*, **47**, 313–4.

RAUSTEN D.S. & OCHS M.A. (1973) Apomorphine-naloxone controlled rapid emesis. *Journal of the American College of Emergency Physicians*, **2**, 44–5.

RAWLINS M.D. (1973) Mechanism of salicylate induced antipyresis. In SCHÖNBAUM E. & LOMAX P. (eds.) *The Pharmacology of Thermoregulation*. Basel, Karger, 311–324.

REDDIN P.C. (1966) Blood Demerol studies. *Journal of the Arkansas Medical Society*, **63**, 187–191.

REVILL S.I., ROBINSON J.O., ROSEN M. & HOGG M.I.J. (1976) The reliability of a linear analogue for evaluating pain. *Anaesthesia*, **31**, 1191–8.

RIDING J.E. (1960) Post-operative vomiting. *Proceedings of the Royal Society of Medicine*, **53**, 671–5.

ROE B.B. (1963) Are postoperative narcotics necessary? *Archives of Surgery*, **87**, 912–5.

ROLLASON W.N. & SUTHERLAND J.S. (1963) Phenoperidine (R1406) A new analgesic. *Anaesthesia*, **18**, 16–22.

ROLLMAN G.B. (1976) Signal detection theory assessment of pain modulation. A critique. *Advances in Pain Research and Therapy*, 1. New York, Raven Press, 355–362.

ROQUES B.P., GARBAY-JAUREGUIBERRY C., OBERLIN R., ANTEUNIS M. & LALA A.K. (1976) Conformation of Met-enkephalin determined by high field PMR spectroscopy. *Nature*, **262**, 778–9.

DI ROSA M., GIROUD J.P. & WILLOUGHBY D.A. (1971a) Studies of the mediators of the acute inflammatory response induced in rats in different sites by carrageenan and turpentine. *Journal of Pathology and Bacteriology*, **104**, 15–29.

DI ROSA M. PAPADIMITRIOU J.M. & WILLOUGHBY D.A. (1971b) A histopathological and pharmacological analysis of the mode of action of non steroidal anti-inflammatory drugs. *Journal of Pathology and Bacteriology*, **105**, 239–256.

RUMACK B.H. & TEMPLE A.R. (1974) Lomotil poisoning. *Pediatrics*, **53**, 495–500.

RUSSELL B. (1959) My philosophical development. London, George Allen & Unwin, 26.

SAMTER M. & BEERS R.F. (1968) Intolerance to aspirin. Clinical studies and consideration of its pathogenesis. *Annals of Internal Medicine*, **68**, 975–983.

SAUNDERS C. (1966) Clinical evaluation of analgesic drugs. *Acta Anaesthesiologica Scandinavica. Supplement XXV 327–9*.

SCRAFANI J.T. & CLOUET D.H. (1971) Biotransformations. In CLOUET D.H. (ed.) *Narcotic Drugs. Biochemical Pharmacology*. New York, Plenum Press, 137–158.

SEED J.C. (1965) A clinical comparison of the antipyretic potency of aspirin and sodium salicylate. *Clinical Pharmacology and Therapeutics*, **6**, 354–8.

SEED J.C., WALLENSTEIN S.L., HOUDE R.W. & BELLVILLE J.W. (1958) A comparison of the analgesic and respiratory effects of dihydrocodeine and morphine in man. *Archives Internationales de Pharmacodynamie et de Thérapie*, **116**, 293–339.

SETTIPANE G.A., CHAFEE F.H. & KLEIN D.E. (1974) Aspirin tolerance. II. A prospective study in an atopic and normal population. *Journal of Allergy and Clinical Immunology*, **53**, 200–4.

SEVELIUS H., MCCOY J.F. & COLMORE J.P. (1971) Dose response to codeine in patients with chronic cough. *Clinical Pharmacology and Therapeutics*, **12**, 449–455.

SEWARD E.H. (1949) Self administered analgesia in labour. *Lancet*, **ii**, 781–3.

SEWELL R.D.E. & SPENCER P.S.J. (1977) The role of biogenic amines in the actions of centrally acting analgesics. In ELLIS G.P. & WEST G.B. (eds.) *Progress in Medicinal Chemistry, 14*. Amsterdam, Elsevier/North Holland Biomedical Press, 247–283.

SEYMOUR-SHOVE R. & WILSON C.W.M. (1967) Dependence on dextromoramide. *British Medical Journal*, **i**, 88–90.

SIEGEL S. (1956) Non parametric statistics for the behavioural sciences. New York, McGraw-Hill.

SIMPSON B.R., SEELYE E., CLAYTON J.I. & PARKHOUSE J. (1962). Morphine combined with tetrahydroaminocrine for post operative pain. *British Journal of Anaesthesia*, **34**, 95–101.

SJÖLUND B. & ERIKSSON M. (1976) Electro-acupuncture and endogenous morphines. *Lancet*, **ii**, 1085.

SMITH G.M., EGBERT L.D. & BEECHER H.K. (1966) The submaximal effort tourniquet method of producing experimental pain in man: Sensitivity to 5 mg of morphine and 0·6 g. of aspirin. *Federation Proceedings*, **25**, 501.

SMITH J.B. & WILLIS A.L. (1971) Aspirin selectively inhibits prostaglandin production in human platelets. *Nature*, **231**, 235–7.

SMITH M.J.H. & SMITH P.K. (1966) The Salicylates: A critical bibliographic review. New York, Interscience Publishers.

SNYDER S.H. & PERT C.B. (1975) Regional distribution of the opiate receptor. In SNYDER S.H. & MATTHYSSE S. (eds.) *Opiate Receptor Mechanisms*. Cambridge (Mass), MIT Press, 35–38.

STOCKMAN R. (1913) The action of salicylic acid and chemically allied bodies in rheumatic fever. *British Medical Journal*, **i**, 597–600.

STONE V., MOON W. & SHAW F.H. (1961) Treatment of intractable pain with morphine and tetrahydroaminacrine. *British Medical Journal*, **i**, 471–3.

SWAIN H.H. & SEEVERS M.H. (1974) Evaluation of new compounds for morphine-like physical dependence in the rhesus monkey. *Bulletin Problems of Drug Dependence*, 36, *Addendum*, 1168–1195.

SWINSCOW T.D.V. (1976) Statistics at square one. London. *British Medical Association.*

TAKEMORI A.E., KUPFERBERG H.J. & MILLER J.W. (1969) Quantitative studies of the antagonism of morphine by nalorphine and naloxone. *Journal of Pharmacology and Experimental Therapeutics*, 169, 39–45.

TAMMISTO T., JÄÄTTELÄ A., NIKKI P. & TAKKI S. (1971) Effect of pentazocine and pethidine on plasma catecholamine levels. *Annals of Clinical Research*, 3, 22–9.

TAUB A. (1974) Floor discussion: Pain threshold. In BONICA J.J. (ed.) *Advances in Neurology. Volume 4: International Symposium on Pain.* New York, Raven Press, 125–126.

TELFORD J. & KEATS A.S. (1961) Narcotic–narcotic antagonist mixtures. *Anesthesiology*, 22, 465–484.

THOMAS K.B. (1964) Reduction of suxamethonium muscle pains. *British Medical Journal*, i, 1639–1940.

THOMSON J.S. & PRESCOTT L.F. (1966) Liver damage and impaired glucose tolerance after paracetamol overdosage. *British Medical Journal*, ii, 506–7.

THORPE M.H. (1966) Tibial Pressure Algesimetry. The significance of changes in pain threshold with reference to the assessment of analgesia. *British Journal of Anaesthesia*, 38, 198–206.

VANE J.R. (1971) Inhibition of prostaglandin synthesis as a mechanism of action of aspirin-like drugs. *Nature*, 231, 232–5.

VAN REE J. (1977) Multiple brain sites involved in morphine antinociception. *Journal of Pharmacy and Pharmacology*, 29, 765–7.

VAN REE J.M., DEWIED D., BRADBURY A.F., HULME E.C., SMYTH D.G. & SNELL C.R. (1976) Induction of tolerance to the analgesic action of lipotropin C-fragment. *Nature*, 264, 792–3.

VEREBEY K., VOLAVKA J. & CLOUET D. (1978) Endorphins in psychiatry. *Archives of General Psychiatry*, 35, 877–888.

VILLARREAL J.E. & SEEVERS M.H. (1972) Evaluation of new compounds for morphine-like physical dependence in the rhesus monkey. *Bulletin Problems of Drug Dependence*, 34, *Addendum* 7, 1040–1053.

WANG S.C. (1963) Emetic and antiemetic drugs. In ROOT W.S. & HOFMANN F.G. (eds.) *Physiological Pharmacology II (part B).* New York, Academic Press, 255–328.

WANG S.C. & GLAVIANO V.V. (1954) Locus of emetic action of morphine and hydergine in dogs. *Journal of Pharmacology and Experimental Therapeutics*, 111, 329–334.

WATERFIELD A.A., HUGHES J. & KOSTERLITZ H.W. (1976) Cross tolerance between morphine and methionine-enkephalin. *Nature*, 260, 624–5.

WAY E.L. (1968) Distribution and metabolism of morphine and its surrogates. *Research Publications of the Association for Research in Nervous and Mental Disease*, 46, 13–31.

WAY E.L. & ADLER T.K. (1962) The biological disposition of morphine and its surrogates. Geneva, World Health Organisation.

WAY E.L., TAKEMORI A.E., SMITH G.E., ANDERSON H.H. & BRODIE D.C. (1953)

Toxicity and analgesic activity of some congeners of salicylamide. *Journal of Pharmacology and Experimental Therapeutics*, **108**, 450–460.

WEI E. & LOH H. (1976) Physical dependence on opiate like peptides. *Science*, **193**, 1262–3.

WEINSTEIN S.H., PFEFFER M., SCHOR J.M., FRANKLIN L., MINTS M. & TUTKO E.R. (1973) Absorption and distribution of naloxone in rats after oral and intravenous administration. *Journal of Pharmaceutical Sciences*, **62**, 1416–9.

WEINSTOCK M. (1971) Sites of action of narcotic analgesic drugs: Peripheral tissues. In CLOUET D.H. (ed.) *Narcotic Drugs, Biochemical Pharmacology*, pp. 394–407. New York, Plenum Press.

WERLE E. (1972) On endogenous pain producing substances with particular reference to plasmakinins. In PAYNE J.P. & BURT R.A.P. (eds.) *Pain: Basic Principles—Pharmacology—Therapy*. London, Churchill Livingstone, 86–92.

WIEGAND R.G. & PERRY J.E. (1962) Absorption of salicylate and acetylsalicylate following oral dosage. *Pharmacologist*, **4**, 154.

WILLOUGHBY D.A., WRIGHT V. & TURNER P. (1977) Proceedings of a symposium on diflunisal—February 1977. *British Journal of Clinical Pharmocology*, 4, Supplement 1. 1S–52S.

WINDER C.V. (1959) Aspirin and algesimetry. *Nature*, **184**, 494–7.

WINTER C.A. (1965) The physiology and pharmacology of pain and its relief. In DESTEVENS G. (ed.) *Analgetics, Volume 5, Medicinal Chemistry*. New York, Academic Press, 10–74.

WOOD P.H.N. (1963) Studies of occult bleeding caused by salicylates and related compounds. In DIXON A. ST. J., MARTIN B.K., SMITH M.J.H. & WOOD P.H.N. (eds.) *Salicylates: An International Symposium*. London, J. & A. Churchill Ltd., 194–198.

WOODBURY D.M. & FINGLE E. (1975) Analgesic-antipyretic, antiinflammatory agents and drugs employed in the therapy of gout. In GOODMAN L.S. & GILMAN A. (eds.) *The Pharmacological Basis of Therapeutics*. New York, Macmillan Publishing Co., Inc., 338.

WOOLFE G. & MACDONALD A.D. (1944) The evaluation of the analgesic action of pethidine hydrochloride (demerol). *Journal of Pharmacology and Experimental Therapeutics*, **80**, 300–7.

WRIGHT N. & PRESCOTT L.F. (1973) Potentiation by previous drug therapy of hepatotoxicity following paracetamol overdosage. *Scottish Medical Journal*, **18**, 56–8.

ZOTTERMAN Y. (1972) A brief review of electrophysiological studies of cutaneous nerves. In PAYNE J.P. & BURT R.A.P. (eds.) *Pain: Basic Principles—Pharmacology—Therapy*. London, Churchill Livingstone, 4–15.

Index